# Kinesiology
# Taping for Dogs

Also by Katja Bredlau-Morich

Kinesiology Taping for Horses

Katja Bredlau-Morich

# Kinesiology Taping for Dogs

The Complete Guide to Taping for Canine Health and Fitness

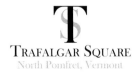

TRAFALGAR SQUARE
North Pomfret, Vermont

First published in the United States of America in 2020 by
Trafalgar Square Books
North Pomfret, Vermont 05053

Originally published in the German language as *Kinesiologisches Taping für Hunde* by **Kynos Verlag, Dr. Dieter Fleig GmbH, Konrad-Zuse-Straße 3, D-54552, Nerdlen/Daun**

**Disclaimer of Liability**

The authors and publisher shall have neither liability nor responsibility to any person or entity with respect to any loss or damage caused or alleged to be caused directly or indirectly by the information contained in this book. While the book is as accurate as the authors can make it, there may be errors, omissions, and inaccuracies.

**ISBN: 978 1 64601 0226**
**Library of Congress Control Number: 2020944757**

All photographs by Robert Bredlau
Book design by Kynos Verlag
Cover design by RM Didier
Index by Andrea M. Jones (www.jonesliteraryservices.com)
Typefaces: Warnock, Bahrim, Agenda

Printed in the United States of America

10 9 8 7 6 5 4 3 2 1

*For Maja,*
*the greatest dog in the world!*

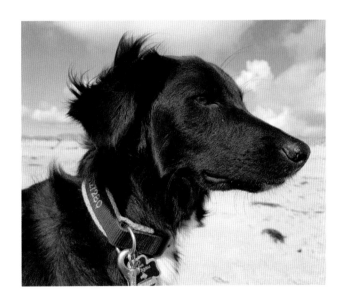

# Contents

## Chapter 5
Various Taping Applications

## Chapter 6
Case Studies from My Physiotherapy Practice

# Preface

Dear Reader,

For several years now, kinesiology taping has been a big component of my daily work as an animal physiotherapist. Again and again, I have answered questions from clients—dog owners and horse owners—about how kinesiology tape works, what it does for animals, and how it affects their bodies. And I was encouraged to write a book because I could explain kinesiology taping in an easy-to-understand way.

In August 2016, my book *Kinesiologisches Pferdtaping* was published, in Germany, followed by the English version *Kinesiology Taping for Horses* published by Trafalgar Square Books in January 2018. As soon as these books were published, dog owners and colleagues working as canine physiotherapists started asking me if, and when, there would be a book for dog taping.

At that point I was excited that I'd managed to write a book for horses. And now, another one?

In order to write a book I need a lot of quiet, patience, and leisure. In my everyday business with animal physiotherapy, tape distribution, preparation and hosting of taping courses, organizing the animal physical therapy convention, and of course, my family, leisure is something that is often non-existent.

But sometimes it all comes together: on the one hand, you just need to hear the questions about a dog-taping book often enough (constant dripping wears even on a stone!), and on the other hand, leisure eventually arrives and the much-needed window of time opens up.

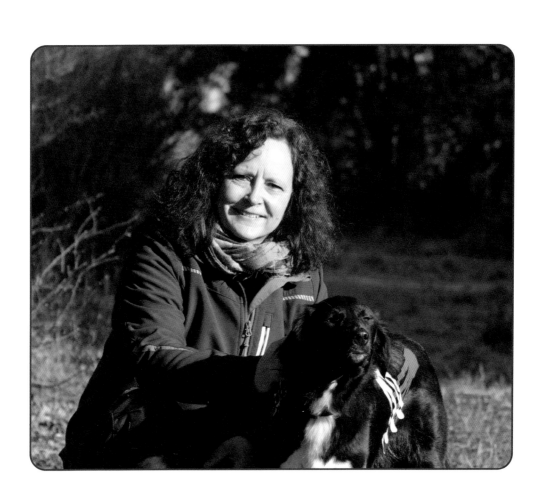

An essential part in the writing of this book is certainly due to our new dog, who came into our lives in the fall of 2018 and who was always looking at me expectantly. In the winter and spring of 2019 I finally found the time and started to write the German version of *Kinesiologisches Taping für Hunde*, which was published that autumn, and Trafalgar Square Books immediately took an interest in publishing the English version, which you are now holding in your hands.

Have fun reading!
Katja Bredlau-Morich
Certified Animal Physiotherapist

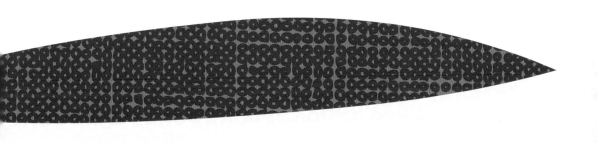

# Chapter 1:
# Basic Information,
# Material, How the
# Tape Works

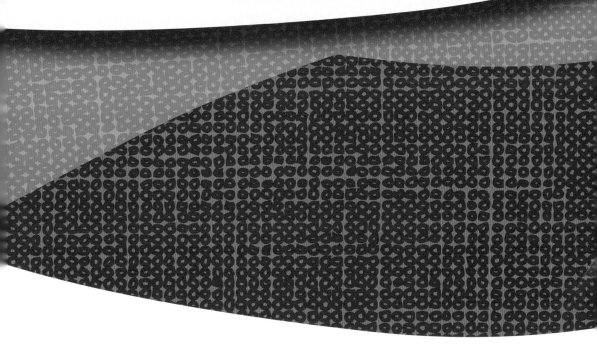

# History and Development of Kinesiology Tape

Like so many other treatments and modalities in the animal industry, kinesiology taping was not originally designed for use on animals. It was primarily developed for use on people. But it proved to be so successful in treating human ailments that over the years kinesiology taping has been adapted for treating animals, as well.

In the 1970s, Dr. Kenzo Kase, a Japanese human chiropractor, had the idea of developing kinesiology tape. He often felt that his treatment of patients didn't last as long as he would

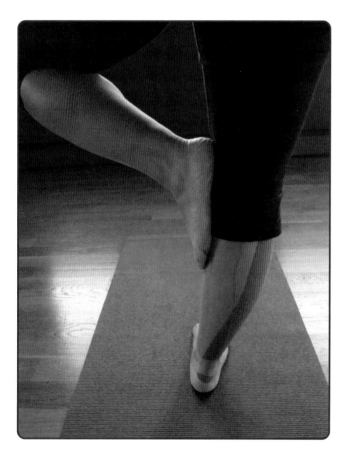

*An athlete with a muscle taping to activate the m. gastrocnemius during a workout.*

have liked. Due to muscle memory and habitual movement patterns, health problems often reoccurred. This is why Dr. Kase was searching for a way to increase the longevity of his chiropractic treatments and enhance the primary effects of his work.

In the 1970s, taping was a treatment modality used quite often. But before kinesiology tape was invented, common athletic tape was used. This kind of tape was very firm and inelastic. It was primarily used to stabilize weak body parts, immobilize them, and restrict movement. In the case of a twisted ankle, the athletic tape was used to keep the ankle still and immobilized. Sprained and bruised fingers were stabilized with this tape by wrapping them together with the fingers next to them. In these cases, athletic tape is still commonly used today.

But that wasn't what Dr. Kase had in mind. He was looking for a material that would support the tissue but move with the body and not restrict the range of motion. Based on his experience, immobilizing and keeping the tissue at a still point was not always the best way to treat a soft-tissue injury.

As opposed to a solid cast for a broken bone, we now know that a certain amount of controlled, light movement is better and more helpful for the healing and regeneration of soft-tissue lesions. Tendons, ligaments, and even muscles do need a certain amount of light, physiological movement during the regeneration process. This gives the newly built body cells an impulse in the direction their growth is needed. Otherwise, you can have disorganized cell growth and development, where the cells don't know in which direction to grow and how they are supposed to work.

With these thoughts in mind, Dr. Kase developed a stretchable, elastic material that would cling to the patient's body surface. Due to its stretchiness, kinesiology tape can move with the tissue without restricting the range of motion of the body. Depending on its application, you can activate or relax a muscle and loosen fascia adhesions, but also support joints like the knee or elbow, yet it doesn't lead to movement restriction in the joints, fascia, or muscles. Human physiotherapists often call kinesiology tape a "second skin" because it adapts so perfectly to motion, while supporting and even enhancing and improving movement patterns.

In addition to all these thoughts, Dr. Kase longed for a treatment modality that had a long-lasting effect on his patients, something they could "take home" with them. This is now possible with kinesiology tape because it can be applied after a chiropractic session and the patient can go home and wear it for several days while the tape is doing its job. Normal everyday activities do not bother the tape: you can wear it at work, while doing all kinds of sports, taking a shower, and so on.... For both humans and animals, a period of four to five days is recommended for a taping-application duration unless it falls off by itself or you have the feeling that the effect is wearing off (more about this later in the book).

As said before, Dr. Kenzo Kase developed this tape during the 1970s. It is difficult to settle on the exact date because such a development often takes a long period of time—from creating the material and adhesive, to studying the effects of the tape and

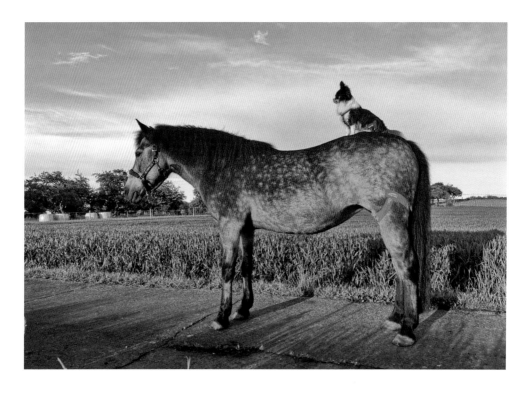

*A Chihuahua and a German sport pony, both with a Knee-Sling Taping to stabilize the knee joint.*

gathering case studies and experiences, to mass production, development of products such as this can be very time consuming. The first time you would have seen kinesiology tape in the general public was in the 1980s during sports events. Back then, a few Japanese and Chinese athletes were wearing the colorful tape strips during athletic competition. But the real breakthrough came with the 2008 Olympic Games, where multiple athletes from various countries used kinesiology tape during their contests. At the 2012 Olympic Games, there were hardly any competitors *not* wearing the colorful tape.

From there it was only a small step before kinesiology tape was widely used in the offices of doctors and therapists everywhere. And because it was working so well for human patients, the next logical step was the taping of animals. The most common animals to be taped are horses, cows, and dogs, but of course you can treat nearly any other animal with it as well. There are also taping applications for cats, guinea pigs, and rabbits.

Many animals engage in athletic performance, like sport horses or agility dogs, while others suffer from arthritis, malformations, or other physical ailments. These animals are treated by veterinarians and therapists (such as physiotherapists, chiropractors, or osteopaths), and the use of kinesiology tape is advisable and helpful in many cases.

## What Does "Kinesiology" Mean?

Before going into detail about the possibilities of application, the name of the tape should be explained in more depth. Where does this term come from and what does it mean?

Kinesiology derives from two Greek words: *kinesis* meaning "motion" or "movement," and *logos* is the Greek word for "word" as well as "study." So kinesiology is the "study of movement." This breaks down into two sub categories: *practical* kinesiology and *medical-scientific* kinesiology.

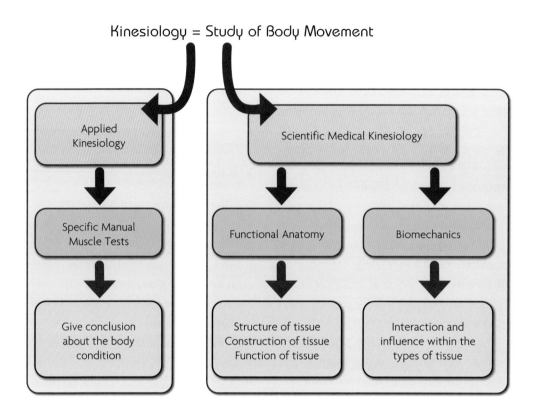

**Applied Kinesiology**
↓
**Specific Manual Muscle Tests**
↓
**Give conclusion about the body condition**

**Scientific Medical Kinesiology**
↓
**Functional Anatomy** / **Biomechanics**
↓
**Structure of tissue Construction of tissue Function of tissue** / **Interaction and influence within the types of tissue**

*The different categories of kinesiology.*

Practical kinesiology is an independent analysis and treatment method in which specific manual muscle tests are done to diagnose muscle tone. With these tests, experienced therapists are able to come to conclusions about the functional state of the body.

Medical-scientific kinesiology, also known as the study of motion, deals with muscles, tendons, ligaments, and bones, and their movement, effect, interaction, and how they influence each other and depend on each other. Since everything is connected in the body, a big focus is placed on the holistic observation of the living being. The study of motion has a huge influence on physiotherapy and rehabilitation of disturbed movement.

Medical-scientific kinesiology itself has two other subcategories, which are *functional anatomy* and *biomechanics*. *Functional anatomy* puts the focus on the structure of the tissue, the motion apparatus, and the organism, as well as the construction, function, and connection of the various tissue types.

The focus of the *biomechanics* is about the interaction of these various aforementioned structures and how movement affects these tissues.

## Terminology: Tape = Tape?

Sometimes you read or hear the term "physio tape." This is practically the same as kinesiology tape in regards to application and effect. It was just named differently by one company to differentiate their product from others. But the term or name started spreading so that today the terms "kinesiology tape" and "physio tape" are used equally, although the tape is basically the same.

I mentioned "athletic tape" in the beginning. This tape is different because it is very rigid, sturdy, and inelastic. It has a different function. It immobilizes and stabilizes the affected area.

And then there is also "dynamic tape," which is made up of artificial fibers and material and is a lot more stretchable than kinesiology tape. It works with massive mechanical retraction forces, and is used on human patients for posture- and body-position correction. Because of its extreme elasticity and huge recoil, animals do not tolerate it very well.

# Kinesiology Tape—
# A Unique Material

## Material

Kinesiology tape is made of a tightly woven cotton fabric, kind of like a T-shirt or a kitchen towel. What makes it so unique are the elastic fibers that are threaded through it in the longitudinal direction of the tape. This is why it is elastic and stretchable in this direction. Because there are no elastic fibers running crosswise, you can't stretch it laterally. This is important to keep in mind when taping small dogs. In these cases, you often need rather small and short strips of tape and you may be tempted to cut them across the roll of tape and not along the tape. Once you try to tear the paper backing off a strip of tape that is cut across, you will see that this isn't possible and there is no vertical stretch to the tape.

## Elasticity

Like a Band-Aid®, kinesiology tape is applied onto a paper backing. With the tape attached to the paper, it is already 10 percent pre-stretched. All brands of kinesiology tape produce their tape this way to prevent wrinkles and an uneven tape. So the tape is pre-stretched lightly (10 percent) so that it is applied evenly and wrinkle-free on the paper backing.

The fact that the tape comes off the paper with this pre-stretch is very important and should always be remembered and taken into consideration when taping animals. In a lot of cases, this 10 percent pre-stretch is as much as you will need; when it comes to animals, most receptor cells are located directly under the skin, around the root of the hair. This is why dogs, horses, cats, cows, rabbits, and all other hairy or furry animals have so much more sensation over their hair or fur than we humans do with our naked skin.

Every manufacturer has their own specifications about the elasticity of their kinesiology tape and it usually varies between 140 percent and 180 percent from the original unstretched length. The various degrees of stretch can be visualized nicely with a tape that has a pattern or logo on it. The more stretch a tape strip has, the more distorted the pattern or logo appears.

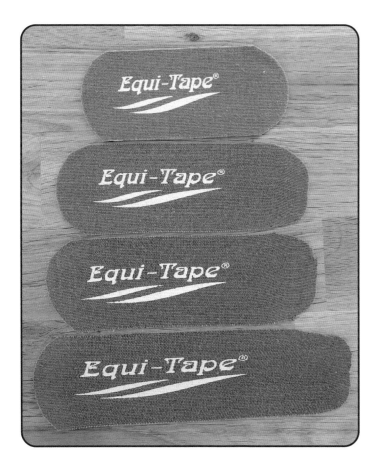

*The various degrees of stretch of four equally long strips of tape. From top to bottom:*
- *No stretch*
- *Light stretch (10 percent off paper stretch)*
- *Medium stretch*
- *Strong stretch*

## Adhesive

A special acrylic adhesive is applied to the back of the tape. This adhesive is llatex-free and medication-free. If you take a closer look at it, you can see that it has a special wave pattern with small adhesive-free intervals. These allow the material to be water- and air-permeable, which highly increases the comfort of the kinesiology tape when applied. A regular Band-Aid® has a complete, closed layer of adhesive (no gaps). After wearing the Band-Aid® for a while the skin underneath doesn't feel and look as healthy anymore: it turns white and very soft and often macerates over time. This is because a closed layer of adhesive does not allow air contact with the skin and the skin can't "breathe." With kinesiology tape and its gaps in the adhesive layer, this is not going to happen. The skin can breathe and even after several days with the tape on, it still looks and feels healthy.

The wave pattern of the adhesive is there for a reason. The adhesive can simply be applied in straight lines (with

gaps in between), but while developing the tape, the adherence proved to be better when adhesive was applied in a wave pattern (the form of a sine wave). The body of the patient (human or animal) does not always move in a straight line. The long back muscle is a good example of this: The muscle begins at the pelvis bone (origin), then runs parallel on the left and right sides of the spine, and attaches at the base of the head (insertion). When this muscle works in its basic linear way, it is responsible for extension and flexion of the spine. But since humans and animals do not only move in a linear

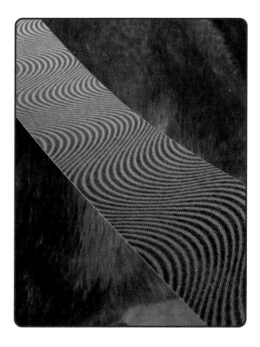

*The back of kinesiology tape with the specific adhesive layer in a "wave" pattern and adhesive-free intervals.*

fashion, the tape needs to be flexible. For example, a dog curls up while sleeping, when he is trying to catch his tail, or when turning in circles. Also, when playing with other dogs he can often twist up like a pretzel! The specific adhesive wave pattern of the sine wave allows the kinesiology tape to move perfectly with the body and compensate for all the shear motions and forces of non-linear movement. It allows the tape to follow all linear and non-linear motions in the best possible way.

The adhesive has one more special feature: It is activated through frictional heat. After applying the tape to the patient, the adhesive is activated by vigorously rubbing over it and thereby releasing its full adherence. This is explained in more detail on page 49.

## Conclusion

It's the combination of the aforementioned characteristics that makes kinesiology tape so special. The cotton fabric, the elastic fibers, and the specific adhesive layer give the tape a skin-like character. This allows the tape to move with the body in every direction. The thickness of the tape is also similar to the thickness of the top layer of skin. Many human patients report that they don't even feel or perceive the tape after a short period of time. Four-legged patients tolerate the tape very well after a short period of acclimatization.

Today there are a lot of different companies producing kinesiology tape in all different colors. Technically, there is no difference in the tape because of the color. That is why these companies always emphasize that it doesn't matter which color tape you buy and use. However, with years of experience, I personally believe that color has quite an impact on the effect of the taping. Color Therapy is a complementary therapy dating back thousands of years. More about colors and their significance can be found on page 19.

A question often asked is: Are all kinesiology tapes the same? Yes and no!

The basic principles, as described already, are always the same, no matter which brand of tape you choose. But depending on the company, the cotton may be woven more tightly or more loosely, the capacity for stretch can be different, and the adhesive may vary quite a lot so that the tape adheres more or less well to the skin or hair.

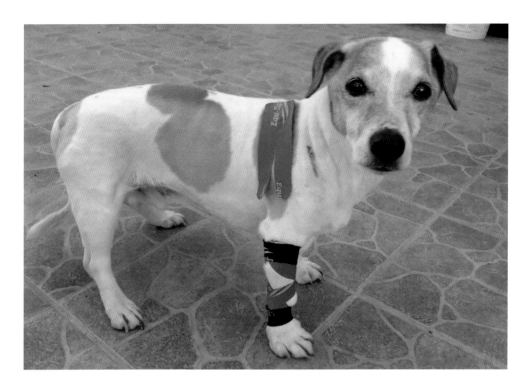

*A Jack Russell Terrier with Muscle
Taping on the shoulder and
Proprioceptive Taping on the front leg.*

Kinesiology tapes developed for people show little to no adhesiveness when it comes to the taping of animals. Here, the tape has to perform much more. Most tapes adhere well to skin, but with hair or fur it is a totally different situation. With animals you have to consider factors such as dirt, dust, mud, and water/humidity. It is not often that a human patient rolls in sand or mud! A dog can get wet in the rain, and sometimes scratch his own hair with his claws and teeth, and maybe scratch the tape as well. Taking this into consideration, some manufacturers have developed special tape for use on animals with a uniquely designed acrylic adhesive. These tapes adhere much better to hair and can cope with the challenge of staying on an animal's coat.

Kinesiology tapes designed specifically for animals are often more expensive than the ones designed for humans.

But there is no benefit when you buy cheap tape, and it doesn't stick well to the hair! Obviously, there is no effect on the dog, and it is frustrating for dog owners and practitioners when the tape appears not to last. That is the point where you often hear, "Oh, this didn't work at all!"

I advise using a specialized kinesiology tape designed for animals even when it is pricier than the more common brand. More about this and the available sizes can be found on page 40.

# How Kinesiology Tape Works

Before we get into more detail about the effects of kinesiology taping and the impact it can have on the body, there is something important to know in advance.

Kinesiology taping is an excellent treatment modality that can induce a lot of good things, but it is not a miracle cure that can solve all problems by itself! In my daily animal physiotherapy work, I use the tape quite often. I would guess that about 75 percent of my patients are sporting colorful stripes after the therapy session.

*But* these taping applications are always applied after a physiotherapy evaluation and treatment. Dr. Kenzo Kase intended kinesiology taping to be an *additional* supportive treatment to enhance and prolong the primary effect of the actual bodywork.

Kinesiology tape, of course, can work by itself. The tape reaches its full potential when the affected tissue (depending on the findings) has been massaged, loosened up, activated, stretched, or mobilized before being taped.

> Kinesiology taping is a supportive treatment modality to be combined with other treatments (such as massage or stretching). It is not a universal miracle cure!

## General Effect

The general effect of kinesiology tape is based on one single, simple, physical rule: everything that is being stretched wants to go back to its natural, unstretched state (neutral position).

It is the same here: when the kinesiology tape is applied to the skin or hair, the stretched material is trying to recoil to its unstretched state. Because it now adheres to the skin or hair, it takes the tissue with it while recoiling, and therefore, pulls the tissue together. This results in the tissue layers being pushed together and lifting slightly, since they have to go somewhere and the only available direction is away from the body. This is called the *lifting effect.*

This *lifting effect* is the basic effect of the tape: it lifts the skin (with animals, it lifts the hair and the upper layer of the skin). This is clearly demonstrated in the picture to the right. But in general, this lifting effect can't be seen since it is at the microscopic level, and when taping humans it can't be seen at all. In the picture here, we purposely overdid it with the amount of stretch so that there would be an extreme recoil and the lifting effect more visible. Please keep in mind that this is a demo picture! In a typical case the hair would be more flat on the body.

The lifting effect leads to more space in the tissue underneath, allowing vessels to dilate, blood and lymphatic fluid to flow more easily, and waste products to be washed out and removed. All of this enhances circulation in the tissue, and therefore, results in a better supply of nutrients, minerals, and oxygen. The lifting effect continues onto the soft-tissue layers underneath,

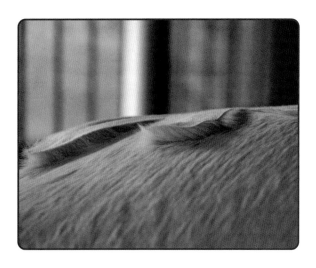

*The tape here was applied with a strong stretch to make the "lifting effect" on hair and skin more visible. Typically, you would not work with this amount of stretch.*

then into the next layer and the next, and works its way through the layers to very deep tissue layers. Therefore, it is possible to reach and influence deeper layers in the body—for example, a *Decompression Taping* (also called *Star Taping* or *Pain Cross*) is often used on dogs suffering from hip arthrosis or hip dysplasia.

Arthrosis itself is, of course, an irreversible process that can't be undone by the tape, and hip dysplasia is not going to disappear. Still, you can help animals by alleviating some of the pain and the side effects. Many times, you can see an immediate improvement in the dog's gait and posture after applying a Decompression Taping.

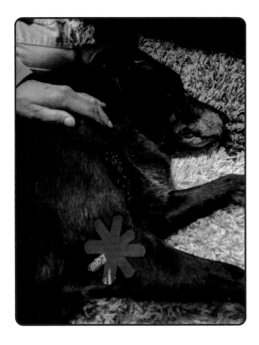

*Decompression Taping for arthrosis in the elbow joint. Through the "lifting effect," deeper parts of the body can be reached.*

## Reduction of Pressure

An increased tissue size is always a result of inflammatory processes, swelling, and painfully tense muscles. Because of this increased size, the pressure in this area increases, resulting in pain.

As described before, kinesiology tape's primary effect is the lifting of tissue, and consequently, creation of space in the affected area. When there is more space, the pressure is taken away from the inflammation, the vessels, and the tight muscles, and this alleviates strain.

## Reduction of Pain

A tight muscle can also be slightly swollen and increased in size because the fibers are in a state of contraction. This swelling causes pressure on the pain receptors in that affected area.

As a result, the already tight muscle can also be painful.

Through the pressure reduction of the tissue mentioned above, the pressure on the pain receptors also lessens, leading to alleviation of pain.

## Improvement of Circulation

When there is swelling in the joints, the extremities, or the torso, and swelling such as hematomas, fluid is accumulated somewhere in the body and can't flow easily anymore. Through the lifting effect of the kinesiology tape, you can create space in, on, and around the swelling. The built-up fluid, whether it is blood or lymphatic fluid, can flow out more easily because the blood and lymphatic vessels are not compressed anymore. In addition, you can use the recoil of the tape to show the built-up fluid a direction to flow out, allowing waste products and pooled lymphatic fluid to be carried away. The build-up will be reduced and removed. The blood—and lymphatic flow—will be improved. This will be explained in more detail in the chapters about *Lymphatic Taping* and *Hematoma Taping* (pp. 74 and 96).

## Support for Joints

Tight, swollen, or blocked joints also find relief and improvement of their functionality through the pressure reduction of the tape.

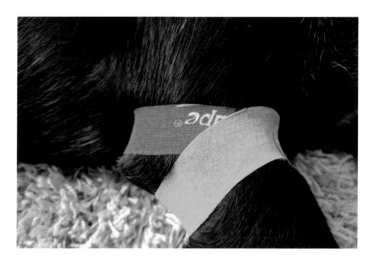

*A Stabilization Taping for the elbow joint.*

Mobility and range of motion will be positively influenced.

Through the skin-like character of kinesiology tape, joints can also be stabilized, depending on the kind of application. Good examples include the knee, the elbow, and the joints of the spine in between the vertebrae without compromising the range of motion of the joints. In the photo on page 16, a *Stabilization Taping* for the elbow joint is displayed. A detailed description of this taping application can be found on page 99—"Stabilization Taping."

## Support of Musculature

Depending on the application, kinesiology tape can either activate or relax a muscle and therefore regulate the muscle tone (see page 66, "Muscle Taping"). Through the direction in which the tape is applied and the direction of the recoil created thereby, muscle contraction or muscle relaxation can be supported.

Besides that, there is improved blood flow in the area of the taped muscle. This leads to a better supply of oxygen, nutrients, and minerals in the area and has a positive effect on muscle activity.

## Improvement of Body Awareness (Proprioception)

Proprioception is described as body awareness and the sense of position of the body and body parts in relation to each other and the surrounding environment. When I close my eyes and move my arm, my brain and my body still know where my arm is and what it is doing—at my side, above my head, flexing the elbow, and so on.

Another example is to close my eyes, take a full glass of water from the table, lift it to my mouth, and drink from it. It will work on the first try, but it could be a little "bumpy." When I repeat this exercise, it gets better and better every time.

Proprioception is based on a sensory system with peripheral receptors called proprioceptors. These are specialized sensory cells, which can be found in all different kinds of tissue—muscle cells, tendons, connective tissue, and also in fascia. Recent studies show that the fascia contains many more proprioceptors than all other tissues, proving again how important it is. These specific receptors give constant feedback to the brain about the condition and tension in the tissue as well as changes therein.

Since the superficial fascia and its proprioceptors—as well as mechanical receptor cells, which react to mechanical impulses like pressure or stretch—are located directly under the skin, they can easily be stimulated with kinesiology tape, and body awareness can be improved.

## Example for the Improvement of Body Awareness

At a trade show, one of the participants came up to me and asked if kinesiology tape could help her dog. He had a successful operation of a disc herniation. The herniated disc had compressed a nerve at the foramen of a vertebra. This led to a dragging of the left hind leg. Even though the operation went well and there was no compression on the nerve anymore, the dog was so used to this gait that he continued to drag the hind leg. I applied a *Proprioception Taping* on this affected extremity. After a few strides, he already showed

improvement in his walk. So I advised the owner to take the dog for a 30-minute walk and when they came back, you could barely see the dragging of the left hind anymore. The disc herniation that had been operated on was not the current cause of the uneven gait; the dog was just used to this movement pattern and stuck in the wrong muscle memory. This example is further detailed in the case studies in chapter 6 (p. 117).

Every taping application influences the body's awareness, but there is a taping application especially designed to address proprioception. More about *Proprioception Taping* on page 110.

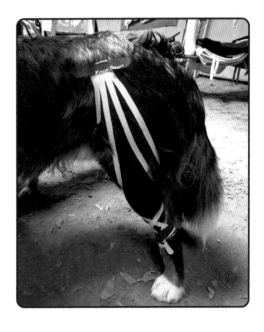

*A Proprioception Taping to improve the body awareness of the left hind leg, caused by a herniated disc operation and gait imbalance.*

# The Colors and Their Significance

Today, kinesiology tape is produced by different companies and brands, and each one has its own variety of colors. According to the manufacturing brands and true to what I've already expressed, there is no objective difference among the tapes because of the color. Within one brand, the tapes are all identical in cotton fabric, fiber thickness, adhesive, and adhesive application. Only the color pigments are different. So why are they produced in different colors?

If the color had no significance at all, it would be totally sufficient to produce kinesiology tape in one single color, especially since most manufacturers state that the colors have no effect.

From the manufacturers' point of view, a full palette of colors is a marketing strategy: A product appeals better to clients when there is a variety of colors to select from.

Nevertheless, there are many practitioners like physiotherapists, osteopaths, and holistic practitioners who believe that there is a difference in the effect of the colors and that the color *does* influence the body.

Medicine has been experimenting with colors since ancient times. Sick people were wrapped in specifically colored blankets, or colored lotions were used. Johann Wolfgang von Goethe was a big believer in color therapy. Many of his writings were about colors and their effect. Color therapy is out there for a reason.

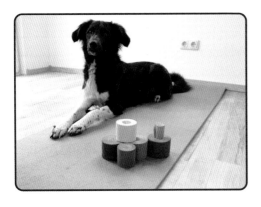

*A variety of different colored kinesiology tapes in the canine physiotherapy office.*

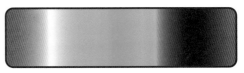

*The color spectrum (light spectrum) goes from infrared to ultraviolet. Every color has a different wavelength.*

From the physical point of view there is a clearly defined spectrum of color that is visible to the human eye—from infrared to ultraviolet. Every color has a specific wavelength within a defined nanometer (nm) range. For example, blue is around 450 nm and red is at 710 nm. Besides that, every color has a specific frequency in the trillion Hertz (THz) range: blue is 650 THz and red is 420 THz.

Considering these different wavelengths and frequencies, a physically different effect on the body's cells seems very likely.

When it comes to taping animals, it is not so much about the optical effect and seeing the tape with their eyes (especially since animals view colors differently than we do), it is more about the physical effect on the body's cells.

## Example of the Effects of Different Colors

At the beginning of my taping practices, I didn't think much about different colors and whether or not they affected treatment. I had a horse patient with a very tight painful back, and I chose the red tape to treat him simply because I liked the color. The application lasted really well on his back, and his pain was quickly alleviated. At the next session, I used blue tape because the horse was a gelding and the color just seemed to suit him. To my surprise, the blue tape did not adhere to the back muscle at all. After a second, very thorough cleaning of the hair, the blue tape still wouldn't stick to the horse. I tried to apply a different roll of blue tape, but that, too, did not stick. So I went back to the red tape (same brand as the blue), and the tape stayed on perfectly.

In accordance with color theory, blue has a cooling effect, while red has a warming effect. When treating a human patient with muscle tension, red light therapy or Fango therapy or heat packs will be used. It seemed that the horse's tight back muscles wanted the warming red tape and not the cooling blue tape.

Nowadays, I usually have eight colors to choose from: red, yellow, pink, blue, black, green, purple, and turquoise. Most of the time, I ask the owners of my four-legged patients if they have a color preference for their animal. Many of them don't care about the color, but there are a lot who instinctively choose the color I would have chosen based on color theory.

## Red

Red is a primary color with dynamic, invigorating, and stimulating qualities.

It raises the energy level, vitality, circulation, and activity. It has a positive effect on the sensory nervous system as well as the metabolism. Red is warming.

Physical data: Wavelength 640–780 nm, Frequency 470–380 THz.

## Yellow

Yellow is also one of the three primary colors. It is stimulating and warming, but not as much as red. It collects and harmonizes energy and has a positive effect on glands and the lymphatic system. The color yellow stimulates the inner organs such as the liver, spleen, gall bladder, stomach, and intestines.

Physical data: Wavelength 570–600 nm, Frequency 530–500 THz.

## Blue

Blue is the third primary color with relaxing and calming properties in a cooling kind of way. It promotes physical relaxation, stress reduction, and a decrease in blood pressure. Because of its cooling and antiseptic qualities, it is often used for treating fever, infections, and sunburns.

Physical data: Wavelength 430–490 nm, Frequency 700–610 THz.

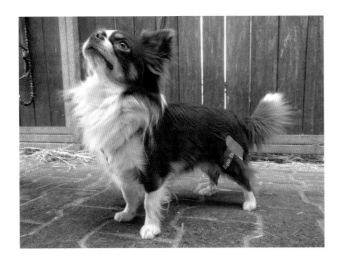

*A Chihuahua is sporting a Knee-Sling Taping to stabilize the knee joint while having a patellar luxation grade I.*

## Pink

Pink is a secondary or mixed color. Depending on the brightness of the color tone, it is said to have gentle and soothing properties. It can bring inner peace and serenity as well as brighten the mood.

Similar to the color red, pink is believed to have an energy-increasing effect.

Physical data: Pink is not part of the classical range of color and is most often declared to be part of the ultra-violet spectrum. Scientifically, it is challenging to find an exact wavelength for this color. Pink is not a color of light found naturally.

## Green

Green is a secondary color, mixed from the colors blue and yellow. It is believed to have the most significant healing, rehabilitative, and relaxing impact. Effects of green can be balancing, harmonizing, neutralizing, and calming. It is often referred to as *the* healing color.

Physical data: Wavelength 490–570 nm, Frequency 610–530 THz.

## Violet/Purple

Violet results from the mixture of red and blue and is, therefore, another secondary color. Its effect is oftentimes a result of the mixture of the contrasting colors red and blue. Depending on the shade, it can either be harmonizing and calming, or energizing. Purple enhances one's concentration.

Physical data: Wavelength 380–430 nm, Frequency 790–700 THz.

## Turquoise

Turquoise is one more secondary color, mixed from the colors blue and green, and believed to strengthen the immune system, stimulate the metabolism, and help fight inflammation. It is also said to have a positive effect on wound healing.

Physical data: Wavelength 500–520 nm, Frequency around 600 THz.

## Black

In the light spectrum, black is not a color. It is more a state of the eye. When no light is reflected into the eye, it sees black. The physical definition of black is the complete absence of color.

Black draws energy from the body and should, therefore, never be used when an animal is in a state of severe fatigue and exhaustion.

Physical data: Since it is not a color, black does not have a defined wavelength or frequency.

I use black kinesiology tape mainly as an anchor to secure the actual taping application and enhance the longevity of a taping application. In this case, the black anchor has little to no physical effect on the body.

On some occasions, I use black tape when there is an animal with a really high energy level. I intentionally use black tape to help calm nervous, fidgety, over-stimulated, and over-excited animals.

You do not have to believe in the effect of colors or incorporate it in your treatment plans to tape successfully. The choice is yours. I have colleagues who are holistic practitioners to whom the right color is essential for the success of their taping application and treatment. Others don't pay attention to this and they tape in pink, simply because they like pink and the way it looks. All people have to decide this for themselves. Personally, my selection is more of a gut feeling. A *Muscle Taping* for a very, very tight muscle will always be taped in red, since red is warming according to color therapy. Through this warming effect, energy is brought to the tight muscle, which is needed for regeneration. With a *Tendon Taping*, on the other hand, I always tape in blue because of its cooling effect. Tendons respond better to cooling.

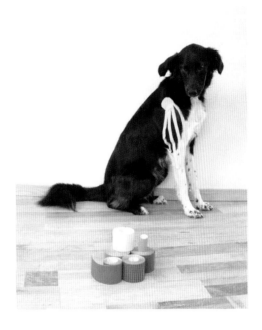

*A Lymphatic Taping on the right front extremity to enhance the lymphatic flow on a slight swelling after a bruise of the elbow joint.*

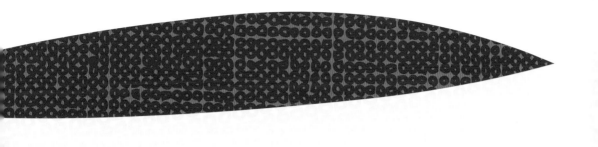

# Chapter 2: Indications and Contraindications

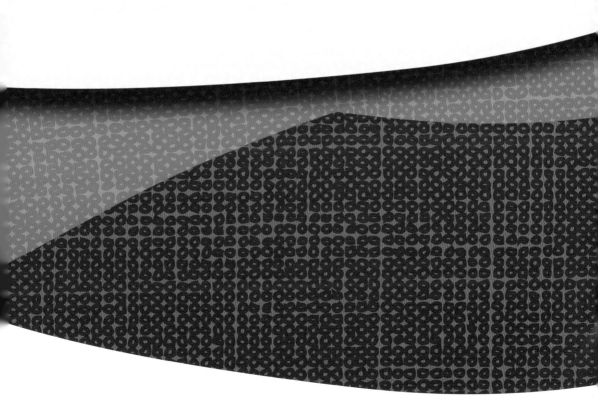

Now that you have taken a closer look at the effects of kinesiology tape, I will focus on problems and situations for which the tape can be used beneficially and where it is not indicated.

Kinesiology tape, in general, is always helpful for any signs of fatigue, after hard work, training, or athletic activities, such as agility competition. Since it helps to improve circulation, it supports the regeneration of muscles after much strain. Improving circulation can also shorten the rehabilitation period.

Since the tape addresses proprioception, body awareness and balance can be improved. Through its skin-like character there is an additional "layer" to the tissue, and depending on the type of application, it can give the body more stability.

# Special Indications

## Muscular Problems

Depending on the kind of strain (or maybe lack of workout), the musculature can be *hypertonic* or *hypotonic, atrophic* or *hypertrophic* (see p. 62). The muscles can be in hard chronic tension or cramping. With the help of kinesiology tape and its lifting effect, blood vessels that serve these muscles will be dilated again. So the blood circulation in the muscles improves and increases, allowing the muscle cells to regenerate more quickly. Depending on the direction of the muscle taping and the recoil that comes with it, you can relax *hypertonic* muscles or stimulate and activate *hypotonic* muscles.

(More about this can be found in the section "Muscle Taping" on p. 66.)

## Fascial Problems

Not only muscular tension can be reduced and regulated with the kinesiology tape; tension in the superficial fascia can also be improved. Fascia covers the muscle tissue as well as the inner organs. These fascia layers sometimes have the tendency to get stuck, and this can disturb the functionality of the tissue underneath of them. With special taping applications, the superficial fascia layers of the muscles can be addressed. These *Fascia Tapings* support the reorganization of the fascia layers and restore their mobility. (More about this can be found in the section "Fascia Taping" on p. 88.)

## Arthrosis

Unfortunately, arthrosis is a problem that can be found quite often in dogs. Genetically caused growth disturbances, acquired body malposition, uneven body balance, or simply too much weight (therefore overloading the bony motion apparatus) can lead to a degenerative restructuring of bones and joints. Even the best tape cannot undo an already existing arthrosis, but it can help reduce the side effects, such as pain. A *Muscle Taping*, for example, can support the muscles surrounding the arthrotic area, and a *Decompression Taping*, with its immense lifting effect, can reduce a lot of pressure in the tissue or the joint, and, thereby, reduce the pain.

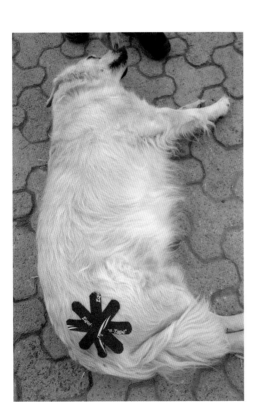

## Swellings

When there is swelling in the leg after an operation or from trauma, a hematoma, or lymphatic swelling, kinesiology tape can activate the circulation and reduce and lessen the swelling. The recoil of the tape supports and enhances the outflow of buildup fluids and waste products. (More about this can be found in the sections "Lymphatic Taping" on p. 75 and "Hematoma Taping" on p. 96.)

*Decompression Taping on chronic hip arthrosis to relieve strain and reduce pain.*

## Joint Instability

One of the effects of the "held-up" tension that comes from some specific taping applications is that kinesiology tape can help support joints without reducing their range of motion. The tape covers the joint like a second skin, giving it additional support without compressing it. Support taping can be suitable for instabilities in the joints of the vertebrae as well as the elbow or knee. (More about this can be found in the section "Stabilization Taping" on p. 99.)

## Trigger Points

With the help of the lifting/decompressing effect of kinesiology tape, trigger points, myogelosis (hardening in the muscle), and localized tight spots in the musculature can find relief through the alleviation of tension. A lot of times these problems can be completely resolved. In most cases a *Decompression Star Taping* should be used, as described on page 92.

## Scar Tissue

Scar tissue can be very rigid and tough and cause motion restriction. You can loosen up scar tissue through the recoil of the kinesiology tape, which encourages the tissue to "relax."

Through the lifting effect, the area around the scar will be supplied with more nutrients, minerals, and oxygen, and the recoil will take away the strain on the scar tissue. But it is a tedious process, and can take some time before scars feel softer and more mobile. In particular, older scars need more sessions of the *Scar Taping* applications. (More about this can be found in the section "Scar Taping" on p. 82.)

## Tendon Injuries, Sprain/ Distortion of the Extremities

Tendon damage and injuries are, unfortunately, a common problem. It is not just extreme athletic activities that can lead to tendon damage. Playing and romping around with other dogs in the field can lead to overstretching, a tear, or even a total rupture of a tendon—yet more situations where the circulatory effect of kinesiology tape can promote the rehabilitation process, and the recoil gives support to the tendon, easing the strain. The damaged tissue is supplied with more oxygen and nutrients through application of the tape, which is helpful for

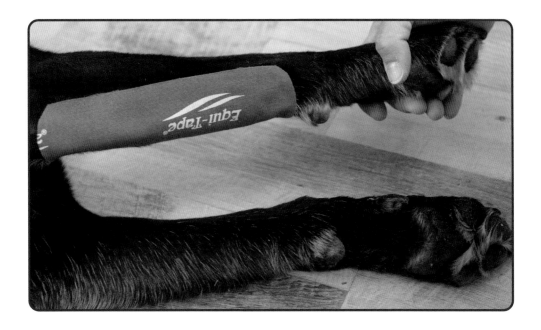

*Tendon Taping on the front extremity with the tape applied from cranial (toward the front/head) to caudal (toward the back/tail) to relieve the strain on an overstretched flexor tendon.*

the regeneration of the injured tendon. (More about this can be found in the section "Tendon Taping" on p. 106.)

## Pain

In general, every taping application has an analgesic (pain-relieving) effect, as a result of the lifting effect and the creation of space that comes with it, the washout of waste products, and the reduction of pressure on the pain receptors. The highest analgesic effect is created by the *Decompression Taping* (see p. 92), which is also called *Pain Cross* because of this specific effect.

# Contraindications

*Contraindication* is a term used to describe a situation in which a procedure should not be used because it may make a treatment risky.

As with most physiotherapy treatments for dogs, kinesiology taping also has indications and situations where the use of the tape is not advised and where you should refrain from using it.

## Direct Contraindications

### Skin Diseases

With a skin disease such as skin fungus, you should refrain from using kinesiology tape and putting it on the afflicted area. Even though it might be helpful for the tissue underneath it (fascia, muscle), the risk of spreading the fungus even further is too high. On the one hand, the fungus could keep on growing and spreading underneath the tape and increase the infected area to encompass other parts of the body, and on the other hand, you have the risk that the practitioner can spread the fungal spores or other germs through simple contact between skin, hair, and tape. The worst case would be spreading it to other parts of the body or even onto other patients. Of course, germs and fungal spores are everywhere around us, but we should not promote further distribution. Hands and scissors can be washed thoroughly after applying the tape. But you can't wash a roll of tape! You cannot avoid contact between the hair of the four-legged patient and a roll of tape, while measuring the length of a tape strip in preparation for the taping application.

### Open Wounds

Open wounds are another instance where you should refrain from using kinesiology tape. Open flesh, blood, and lymphatic fluid would make it difficult for the tape to adhere to this area anyway. Besides, it could have a harmful effect on the healing process. Kinesiology tape enhances circulation, which in this case might not be helpful and could even cause excessive scarring and scar tissue. As soon as a wound is completely healed externally, the scab has fallen off by itself, and stitches have been removed by your veterinarian, you can consider applying a *Scar Taping*. This is helpful when the scar tissue is causing motion restrictions or blocking the energy flow to the affected area.

## Fever

Most physiotherapeutic modalities are designed to enhance circulation and blood flow. This also applies to kinesiology tape. In case of a fever, the body needs all its energy for the immune defense. So when the patient has a temperature, you should refrain from a physiotherapy treatment and a taping application. A fever should be treated by a veterinarian, if necessary, and when the dog's temperature is down again, you can make another attempt at taping.

## Localized Infections

A dog can get a thorn or some other object stuck in his paw, which can cause an infection. In the worst-case scenario, this can cause infection within the whole extremity, which becomes swollen and inflamed. In this situation, a *Lymphatic Taping* application would make sense. *But* as long as there is still an infection and heat in the extremity, *never* apply tape in that region! Because of the circulatory effect of the kinesiology tape, you are at risk of spreading the pathogen further in the body and making the situation worse.

After the infection has been treated and has subsided, if there is still residual swelling, a *Lymphatic Taping* can be applied to help reduce the built-up fluid.

## Pregnancy

It is now quite common for pregnant women to get taped on the abdomen in order to give the connective tissue some support. Of course, they can remove the tape immediately if it is uncomfortable or they feel it isn't working. With dogs, it is slightly different since they are not capable of removing the tape themselves, so you should not tape a pregnant dog. You can never predict what might cause early contractions. That's why it is advisable to keep the risk for mom and pups as low as possible and refrain from using kinesiology tape on the abdomen during pregnancy.

## Malignant Tumors

As described several times before, kinesiology tape enhances circulation. This can have a negative impact on a malignant tumor: increasing circulation can lead to the growth of the tumor itself and also to its spreading within the body. Malignant tumors are an absolute contraindication for taping!

## Hypersensitivity

In my years of using kinesiology tape, I have never seen any sensitivity reactions such as a rash or itching. However, there is always the possibility of an allergic reaction to it or the acrylic adhesive. If this should happen, remove the tape immediately and bathe the dog with warm water.

## Indirect Contraindications

Unfortunately, when it comes to taping dogs, there are two factors that are not, or almost not, important when taping other animals like horses or cows. These are: length of hair and tolerance of the dog. They are not real, direct contraindications, but it is always worth a thought about whether taping is really necessary and beneficial in such cases.

### Length of Hair
The shorter the dog's hair, the better the effect of the kinesiology taping, as well as the results. Tapes that are

*With this length of hair, the tape has little to no effect, because the lifting effect can hardly reach the skin and the receptors within the skin.*

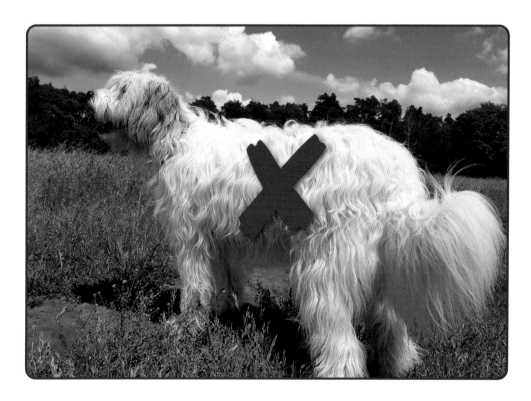

especially designed for taping animals can still adhere to longer hair without any problem. For example, I have taped Australian Shepherd dogs successfully, and the tape stuck very well to the hair. We could see a real improvement in the gait and posture. But when the hair is really long, like an Afghan Hound, for example, it is questionable how much of the lifting effect can actually reach all the way to the surface of the skin. Also, the recoil of the tape will hardly be noticeable, since the hair is too long. The hair will just flip to the other side.

With really longhaired dogs, you should think about how vital the taping application really is because you have to clip the dog's hair in the affected area for a successful taping. This is something all dog owners have to think about and decide for themselves.

### The Dog's Tolerance

This is the second indirect contraindication, which is not as important when taping horses and cows. Ninety-nine percent of large animals do not care about the tape on their hair and tolerate it really well.

With dogs this is a completely different situation. It is the same with bandages: some dogs care little about it, while others almost instantly start chewing it. If your dog is more of the chewing type, it is helpful to keep him busy during the first few minutes after the tape has been applied. Take him for a walk, play with him, or just keep an eye out until the dog gets used to the feel of the tape. Once the dog is used to the tape on his hair, future applications will be tolerated more easily. Most of the time, dogs tolerate the kinesiology tape better than a bandage (under which a painful or itching wound can be found most often). To help the dog acclimate to the tape and prevent him from chewing the material, it's a good idea to put a T-shirt over his abdomen or a sock over the paw or leg, depending where the taping application is located.

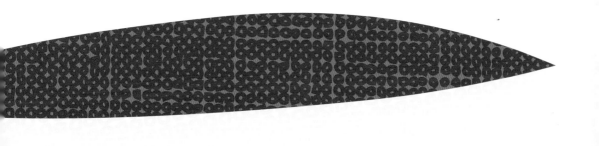

# Chapter 3:
# Handling and
# Practical Application

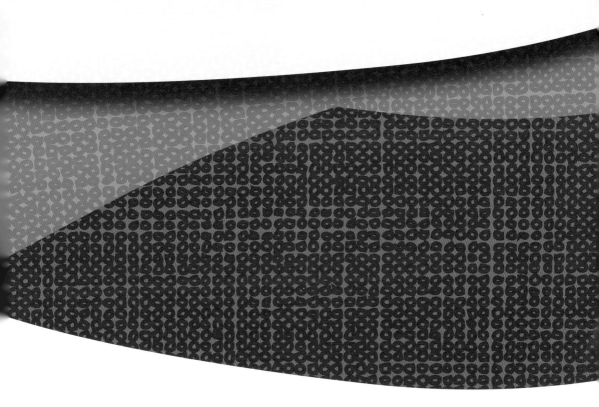

# Preparation of the Dog and His Hair

The dog has to be clean: the tape will not adhere to dust, mud, and dirt, or it can stick to the dirt but not to the hair. When taping over dirt, it might adhere for a short period but will fall off sooner than desired—most likely in combination with the layer of dirt. So it is crucial to brush the dog before the treatment and to remove dust and dirt from the hair.

Another crucial factor is that the dog must be dry; it's not helpful to give the dog a full bath directly before the therapy session. The kinesiology tape does not adhere to wet hair at all! If the dog owner feels that his or her dog is filthy and requires a bath, then he should be bathed the day prior to the taping application so that the hair has a chance to fully dry. Even days with high humidity and rain can make taping more challenging. The dog might seem dry on the top layer of his hair, but humidity often settles in the deeper layers.

Dogs that participate in breed shows are often treated with all kinds of sprays to make the hair shinier; long-haired dogs, whose hair tends to tangle, are treated with a special detangling spray to make it easier to comb.

No matter what kind of spray it is, once applied to the hair, kinesiology tape will not stick anymore! These sprays straighten hair structure and smooth the surface of the hair. Therefore, adherence of the tape to hair that has been sprayed is very poor. You will notice this immediately because kinesiology tape just curls up and rolls off right after the application.

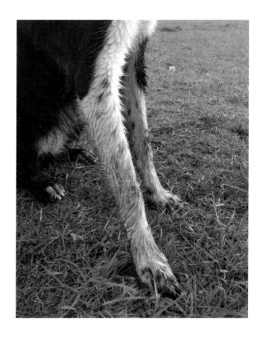

*The tape does not adhere very well to wet or dirty hair. The dog and his hair have to be clean and dry to enable the best adherence so the tape can provide the highest effect.*

# Tricks and Aids to Improve Adhesion

## Clipping the Hair

A question many dog owners ask is whether or not their dogs should be clipped. There is no standard response to this question as it always depends on the length of the hair. Shorthaired dogs like Beagles, Great Danes, or Vizslas definitely don't need to be clipped. Their hair is very short and perfect for a taping application.

For dogs with medium-length hair or curly hair, you just have to give it a try.

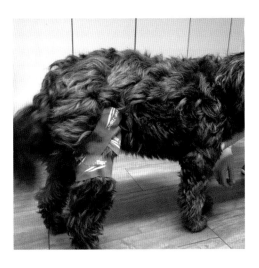

*A hind-leg Sling Tape (p. 103) adheres well even to longer or curly hair. This taping application stayed on for a week.*

I have successfully taped Australian Shepherds, Poodles, and other fuzzy mixed-breed dogs without clipping their hair, and the tape stuck firmly—and you could see the improvement in gait and posture.

As previously mentioned, with really longhaired dogs, clipping the hair is mandatory for the taping application to be beneficial. The recoil can be difficult to achieve with long hair because it will just flip the hair in the other direction.

So if clipping is necessary, choose a length where you do not clip it all the way down to the skin as you would do for an operation, for example. It is better to leave a short layer of hair of about a half-inch (about one centimeter) so that the hair rests flat on the body. Kinesiology tapes especially designed for animals have strong adhesive and very good grip. Removing tape from an animal's bare skin can be really uncomfortable.

If the hair is too short and is sticking up like a hedgehog, the tape will not adhere to it either. This would be like trying to put a Band-Aid® on a hairbrush!

That's why when clipping for a taping application I highly recommend keeping a short layer of hair.

## Spray Adhesive

Every dog breed is different. Along with hair length, some have greasier skin and hair, which also compromises the adherence of the tape. To combat the greasy issue, several companies recommend a special medical adhesive spray. This can be sprayed onto the body part to be taped prior to application to improve the adherence of the tape.

I am not a big supporter of spray adhesive on dog hair. I am very reluctant to spray adhesive on healthy dogs with a healthy hair coat. In fact, at the beginning of my taping career, I bought a bottle of spray adhesive and left it in my car trunk with my other equipment. When I sold the car a few years later, I found the bottle again, still originally sealed and way past the date of expiration!

After my many years of taping animals and lots of experience, I strongly believe that when the tape doesn't stick, there is a reason behind it, no matter what kind of tricks and aids you use. In these cases (which don't happen very often), I always think it's because the body does not want or need the tape. So I change my approach and don't bother that animal with kinesiology tape.

## Baby Powder

If necessary, I use regular baby powder to improve adhesiveness. When the tape doesn't stick due to humidity or greasy/oily skin, I remove the whole application. Then I take regular baby powder and spread some of it over the application area. I rub the powder in gently, and after a few minutes, I thoroughly wipe it away with a cotton or microfiber towel. Microfiber is better because it gets the most powder out of the hair. It is essential to work thoroughly when wiping off the baby powder. Residual baby powder in the hair can stick to the tape and prevent it from adhering. Once the powder is removed entirely and the hair is dry and the skin no longer greasy or oily, the taping applications can adhere much better.

# Does Taping Affect a Dog's Activity?

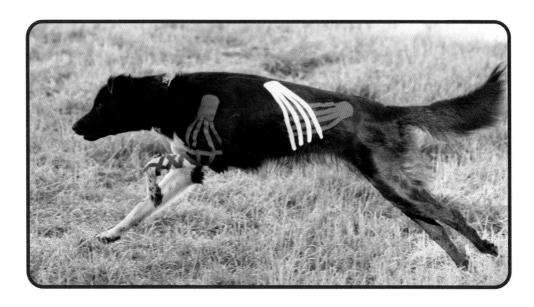

*Kinesiology tape does not compromise movement, and it doesn't restrict daily walks, or playing and romping with other dogs.*

A taped dog can do everything as usual and participate in all his normal activities (swimming included), just like human athletes do by continuing to participate in their sports and maintaining their daily routines. Anything can be done that is not detrimental to their recovering from what made the kinesiology tape necessary in the first place. The same applies to your dog.

An agility dog with a rupture of the cruciate ligament that has been treated with a *Stabilization Taping* or a *Knee-Sling Taping* should refrain from competing until the rupture has healed completely. But, of course, this dog, like any other dog with a cruciate ligament tear, can go for his regular daily walks as recommended by his veterinarian.

You don't have to limit your dog's activity because of the kinesiology tape, but you should be mindful of the injury.

# Preparation and Handling
# of Kinesiology Tape

## Tape Selection

Today there are a variety of brands of kinesiology tape available. Some of them even have so-called "precuts." But these are designed for human patients. There are special precuts for the knee, shoulder, fingers, and back, just to name a few. Unfortunately, the anatomical structures of dogs are different and smaller; therefore, these precuts are of no use when it comes to taping applications for dogs.

So the best thing for dog taping is still the classic tape roll, which is 2

*Today, kinesiology tape for the veterinary service industry is made by different companies, and it comes in various sizes and colors.*

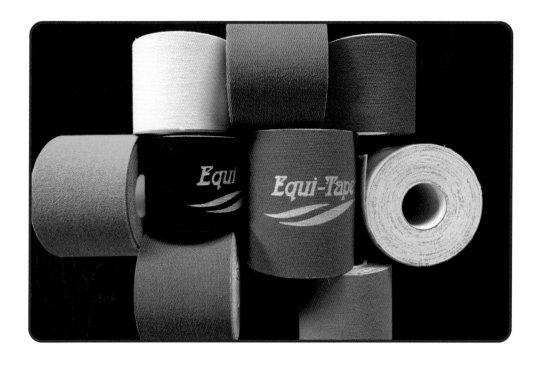

inches (5 cm) wide and about 16 feet (5 m) long.

Within the various brands, there is a lot of difference when it comes to the quality of the tape. Cheap tape often adheres poorly or doesn't stick at all to the hair. It is essential to use a brand of tape specially designed for animal use.

With the use of tape rolls, you can measure directly on the dog, finding the required length of tape needed for the desired taping application, and then cut it to specifications. It is very helpful that almost all brands have lines or grid patterns on the paper backing. This gives you an idea of how long the needed tape strip is, and you can take notes for future applications.

Throughout this book, there are pictures of tape that has the logo Equi-Tape® on it. Fifteen years ago, this was the first tape ever explicitly designed for application on animals. Veterinarians developed it for horses with a special adhesive for application on hair, so it is excellent. Over time it proved not only to work well on horses but also on all other animals with hair, like cows, dogs, and cats. Even though it was developed and named for horses, it can, of course, be used for dogs as well.

There are other veterinary brands, but since their name or logo doesn't indicate that it is for a specific animal, it does not create any confusion. The question, "Is this tape only for horses?" doesn't come up. You have to test them yourself and find which brand and product works best for you and your dog.

## The Right Size

Other factors you have to take into consideration are the different dog breeds, their size, and body shape. A Chihuahua needs smaller and fewer tape strips than a Great Dane. A Doberman Pinscher requires larger-sized tape strips than a Jack Russell. Even among the smaller breeds, there is much variation. The length of tape for a back muscle taping on a Dachshund will most definitely be longer than the one for a Pug. Due to variations in size of different dogs, taking an individual measurement for the length of the needed tape strip is absolutely necessary. Since kinesiology tape was primarily developed for human application, the 2-inch (5 cm) rolls proved to be the best size for the use on two-legged patients. This size is also the perfect width for larger animals such as horses or cows. For dogs, especially smaller dogs, these 2 inches are often too wide. At this time, there are hardly any manufacturers producing smaller tape strips, and it is helpful

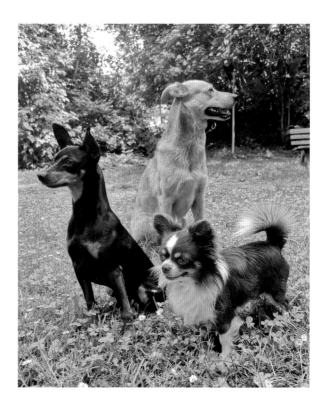

*The variety of dog breeds and the various sizes of animals require an individual measurement of each tape strip to find the right length.*

to cut the tape lengthwise down the middle to make thinner strips.

In an extreme case, like the aforementioned Chihuahua, the tape strips sometimes need to be split lengthwise into four equal segments. NOTE: Never cut the tape crosswise, since it is not stretchable in that direction (see p. 8)!

## Different Tape Shapes

When using kinesiology tape rolls (not precuts), you can cut them into all kinds of shapes and combine them with each other. The most commonly used shapes are the *I-Tape*, the *Y- (or V-) Tape*, and the *Fan-Tape*. There are, of course, more shapes, but they are not used very often. Of course, there is no limitation to your own creativity.

### I-Tape

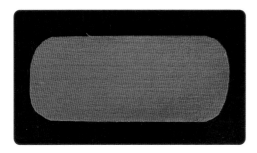

*The I-Tape is a single, straight strip of tape, which has rounded corners on both ends.*

The basic I-Tape is a simple, straight strip of tape, where the edges on both ends are cut to rounded corners. It can be used for both the *End-to-End* technique and the *Inside-Out* technique, which will be described when we get to "Taping Techniques" (p. 44).

### Y- (or V-) Tape

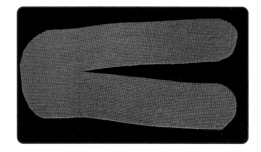

*The Y-Tape or V-Tape has one "closed" end and then splits into two "fingers" at the other end.*

Whether you call this tape cut a Y-Tape or a V-Tape depends on your point of view and on the individual style of cutting it into shape. If you prefer a smaller closed end (also called the "base") it looks more like a "V," as seen in the picture above. But if you like it better with a longer end piece, it looks more like a "Y." That is why this shape has two names.

No matter how you cut it, this shape always has one closed end and then splits into two "fingers." Splitting the tape increases surface coverage. You can better cover a larger area with a Y- (V-) Tape shape. The Y- (V-) Tape cut is always used as an *End-to-End* technique (see p. 44).

## The Fan-Tape

Similar to the Y- (V-) Tape, the *Fan-Tape* has one closed end, but it has multiple fingers. It is up to you how many fingers you cut into it. Some practitioners prefer three fingers, others four, and some go for five fingers on the Fan-Tape.

Here, you also have a surface enlargement by splitting the tape strip in multiple fingers. The more fingers this shape has, the more surface you can cover. The Fan-Tape shape is mostly used for the *Hematoma Tapings* and *Lymphatic Tapings*, when you want to decompress and alleviate a large swollen area on the body or the extremity as quickly as possible. With the Fan-Tape, you always use the *End-to-End* techniques (more on this coming next).

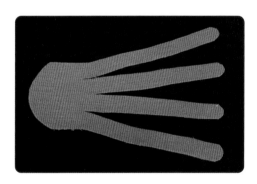

*The Fan-Tape has one closed end and multiple fingers, usually between three and five.*

## Taping Techniques

In general, there are only two techniques for applying the tape onto the patient, which I explain next. How they are applied precisely for each taping application is detailed with step-by-step instructions in the next chapter (see p. 57).

### End-to-End Technique

All Fan-Tapes and Y- (V-) Tape are applied with the *End-to-End* technique. When applying a single I-Tape strip. as in *Muscle Taping*, for example, the *End-to-End* technique is also be used.

This means that you apply a primary end (A) first. When using a Y- (V-) Tape or a Fan-Tape, this is always the closed end. Then the effective area of the tape (B) is laid down, which is either the middle part of a single I-Tape or the fingers of the Y- (V-) Tape, or

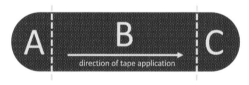

*A schematic presentation of a tape strip that is applied with the End-to-End technique. A = primary end, B = effective area of the tape strip with the direction of taping, C = secondary end.*

Fan-Tape. Then the secondary end (C) is applied. In case of a Y- (V-) Tape or Fan-Tape, these are the endings of the fingers. You are working from one end of the tape strip to the other end.

Since kinesiology tape always recoils toward the primary end (A), the recoil (see definition on p. 14) in the *End-to-End* technique is always directed in the opposite direction from the actual direction of the taping application.

For example, applying a *Muscle Taping* for the long back muscle from cranial (toward the front/head) to caudal (toward the back/tail—see p. 60): The primary starting end (A) is applied cranially (close to the shoulder blade). The effective part of the tape (B) runs parallel to the spine along the muscle. The secondary end (C) is applied caudally, close to the sacrum. The kinesiology tape contracts with its recoil toward the primary end (A) at the shoulder blade.

### Inside-Out Technique

This technique is only used with the application of I-Tapes—for example, with *Decompression Taping, Stabilization Taping* and *Scar Taping.*

With this technique, you don't have a primary end. You tear and remove the paper backing in the middle of the tape strip, and you stretch the tape evenly at both ends, inside-out, and apply it to the patient. The effective area of the tape strip is in the middle. With the inside-out technique, the kinesiology tape recoils from the outside to the center of the tape strip. The ends on the right and left are both secondary ends (C).

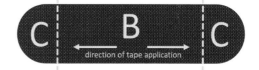

*A schematic presentation of a tape strip that is applied with the Inside-Out Technique. B = effective area of the tape with the direction of taping, C = secondary ends.*

## Scissors

Next to the tape itself, the second most important tool for kinesiology taping is the scissors! Don't save your money on scissors; good ones are essential. Since kinesiology tape is made of cotton fabric, you need an excellent pair of cutting scissors, because it is just like cutting up a T-shirt. Taping scissors are much sharper than regular household or kitchen scissors. Good taping scissor blades also have a titanium coating, which prevents the adhesive from sticking to the blades.

Regular household scissors can only cope with the cutting of kinesiology tape for a short period of time. Not only do they dull quickly, the blades get sticky. This is why you should look for high quality taping scissors right from the beginning. Almost all tape producers have special taping scissors in their equipment section.

## Handling of Kinesiology Tape

### Rounded Corners
As you have seen in the previous pictures, all applied tape strips have rounded corners, even though the

tape comes off the roll with edges. The corners are deliberately cut off and rounded, for the same reason that most Band-Aids® have rounded edges: sharp edges of the tape or Band-Aid® can rub off quicker and unravel faster. Pointed edges may easily get snagged on your fingers, clothes, leash, collar, velcro closures, or a brush or comb. To avoid this, as well as a premature detachment, and to enhance the longevity of the taping application, the corners of the tape are cut off and rounded.

### Removal of the Paper Backing
Once you have measured the right length of tape and cut it into the desired shape, you progress to the next step where you have to remove

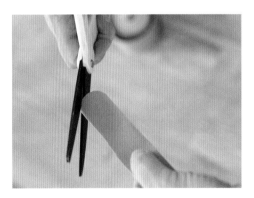

*The corners of the ends of the tape are always cut off and rounded to avoid getting caught on things, and to prevent a premature detachment of the tape.*

### Tip
When you have measured the required length of tape on the dog, you can just fold over the tape at the desired length and cut the rounded corners (see photo). This saves you a little bit of time and it has the advantage that both ends, the one for your tape strip and the one that is still on the roll, get rounded corners with just one cut.

the paper on the backside of the tape and expose the adhesive layer. Please do not fiddle around trying to remove the paper on one end of the tape strip. That is not only tedious, it can also take too long. Instead, just tear the paper backing vertically at the desired point. This is not going to harm the kinesiology tape—it won't fall apart and it also won't wear out or lose its elasticity.

Once you have torn the paper backing vertically, with the paper backing still solidly sticking to the tape, the best thing to do is to pull hard on one end of the tape strip. This causes the paper to detach from the tape at the point where the paper was torn.

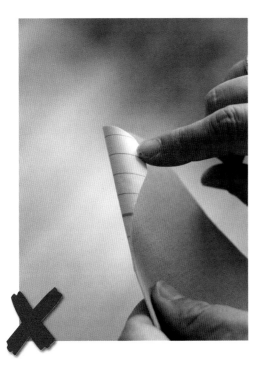

*When removing the paper backing, don't try and fuss with it at one of the corners or edges of the tape strip.*

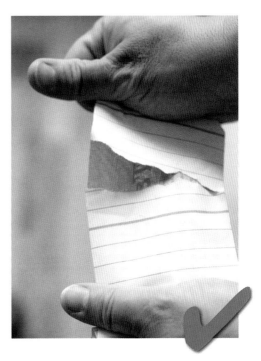

*To remove the paper backing from the tape at a desired spot, tear the paper completely crosswise and unveil the tape.*

## Flat Fingers

Kinesiology tape should always be applied with flat fingers. This makes sure you have an even stretch throughout the whole tape strip, which is highly beneficial for creating the greatest area of effect.

Never use pointed fingers when holding, stretching, and applying the tape. This position will lead to uneven stretch across the width of the tape.

Kinesiology tape will have more stretch in the center where the thumb is stretching the tape (see photo below) than on the upper and lower outer edges of the strip. This unevenness causes an irregular and compromised area of effect within the tape.

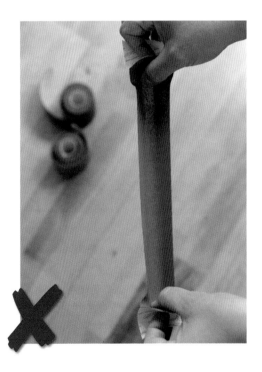

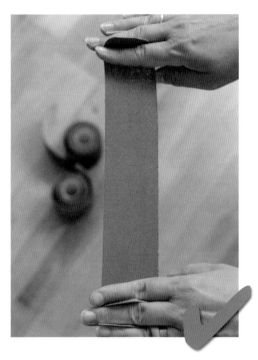

*Do not hold, stretch, and apply kinesiology tape with a single, pointed finger. This will lead to a partial and uneven stretch of the material.*

*When handling the tape, it is important to pay attention to holding it with flat fingers in order to create an even and perfect stretch over the whole width of the tape strip.*

## Stretch-Free Endings

The ends of the tape strip should always be applied with absolutely no stretch to avoid overstretching in the whole application. The more stretch you have at the ends, the more tension you'll get in the whole taping application, increasing the possibility of the tape detaching faster. In addition, it is helpful to push the stretch-free endings (primary and secondary ends) back a little toward the center of the tape strip while applying it. This is known as the "backup."

## Frictional Heat

Another specialty of the adhesive layer is that the adhesive can be activated with heat. Once the entire taping application is applied thoroughly, it is recommended to rub back and forth

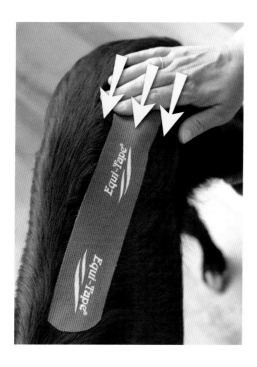

*The ends of the tape strip should always be applied without any stretch. This can be supported with a "backup," demonstrated here with the yellow arrows.*

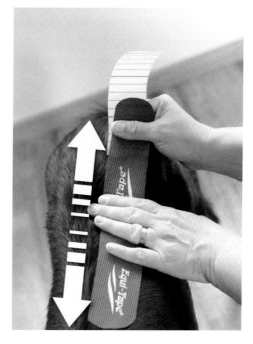

*Rubbing back and forth (see yellow arrow) causes friction, and friction produces heat, which improves the adherence of the tape.*

vigorously but carefully until your hand feels really warm. This will produce frictional heat and through this heat the adhesive on the kinesiology tape will be activated.

In the summer, when it is warm outside, you don't necessarily have to do this. Instead, just let the dog lie in the sun for up to five minutes or take him for a walk in the sun. However, in the winter it is absolutely necessary to rub over the tape to produce the heat. When it is possible, you can let the dog rest under a heat lamp for five minutes in the winter, or put a warm water bottle on him.

## Reusability

Very important: Once kinesiology tape has been applied to an animal, it cannot be reused! This is very important in case of a "misapplication." You can't remove the tape, reposition it, and apply it again. While applying and removing the tape, there is always a small amount of dust, loose hair, and grease sticking to the tape, contaminating the adhesive and thus preventing it from sticking a second time. Human applications also run into the same issue, and it is not practical to use the tape a second time. If you are not satisfied with your taping application because you missed your

target area, there is only one thing you can do: remove the strip of tape, throw it away, cut a new piece, and apply the new one more accurately.

## Removing the Tape

When removing tape from the dog, you should always peel it off in the direction of the hair growth. Some brands

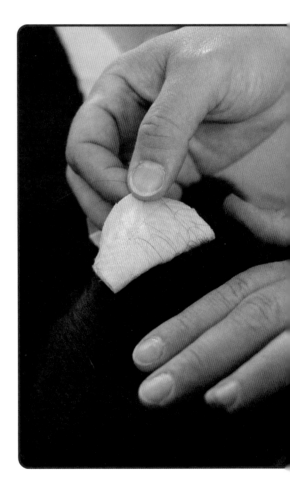

adhere more strongly than others, and the tape should never be yanked off. Aggressive removal of tape can cause an unwanted reaction, especially if you have a sensitive animal. A muscle, for example, that had just been taped to help it relax might involuntarily contract due to the sudden pain caused by a quick pull of the tape. One could claim that in some cases the actual effect of the kinesiology taping is compromised and undone by removing the tape so drastically. It is helpful to take one hand and gently press down on the skin or hair while the other hand is gently pulling off the tape strip. Most pain receptors are located around the roots of the animal's hair. So if you hold on to the hair gently, you can lessen the strain on the roots of the hair and make it less uncomfortable for the dog.

In rare cases, you can find fine lines of adhesive on the hair after removing the kinesiology tape. These can easily be removed with a warm, wet towel.

## How Much Should Tape Be Stretched?

This is one of the most common questions. Some brands and instructional courses refer to the amount of stretch as 10, 20, 50 or 100 percent. I find these terms rather unhelpful. Who is going to stand next to their dog with a ruler or calculator to figure out the right amount of stretch in the strip of tape?

I prefer the terms *light, medium,* and *strong*. Since this is a very subjective feeling—"how much stretch" you have—it takes some practice and experience until you get a sense for the right amount.

I always recommend two things to keep in mind:

*Always remove the tape following the direction of the hair growth. You can use your free hand to hold on to the hair of the dog, to reduce the strain on the roots of the hair and make it less uncomfortable.*

1. The softer the tissue I am working on, the less stretch is needed.

   - Muscle and fascia: light stretch.
   - Tendons and ligaments: light to medium stretch.
   - Bones and joint: medium to strong stretch.

2. The ultimate rule for the right amount of stretch when taping animals is *less is more*!

Too much stretch in the tape always causes too much tension on the hair, the roots of the hair, and the skin underneath it. This can also cause irritation to the pain receptors in that area, which can feel very uncomfortable. Human patients can talk to a therapist and explain how it feels, or even remove the tape themselves when it feels highly unpleasant. Our four-legged patients are not capable of telling us and, depending on the position of the tape, can't remove it by themselves. Too much tension on the tape can lead to unwanted, maybe even aggressive reactions from the dog to the tape. In these cases, the tape should be removed immediately, and you should try to apply it again with noticeably less stretch. It is important to keep an eye on the dog for a while after applying kinesiology tape. Noticeable defense reactions, such as running or rolling to get away from the tape, trying to chew on it, or get it off, are responses to too much tension in the tape and are often immediately indicated by the animal.

A classic beginner's mistake is to work with too much tape stretch. But since it is so stretchy, one is always trying to get as much out of it as possible. I did the same thing in the beginning and I can see this happening a lot of times in my taping courses. In this case, it is helpful to tape yourself occasionally. Cut three equally long strips of tape and apply them with different amounts of stretch on your upper leg, for example: the first strip with the 10 percent off-paper stretch, the second with medium stretch, and the third with very strong stretch. Usually, it only takes a few seconds before the tape strip with the strong stretch is identified as the one that feels the most uncomfortable.

Even taping applications like *Proprioception Taping*, which are applied with no stretch at all, have an effect, and they influence the body awareness in the taped area.

> Always remember that kinesiology tape comes with a 10 percent pre-stretch on the paper backing. These 10 percent are often enough stretch when taping dogs.

## Anchors

Anchors are single I-strips, which are commonly applied at the beginning or end of a taping application, perpendicular to it and with no stretch. They don't have any influence on the actual taping application, except giving

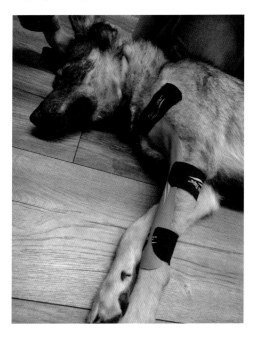

additional "anchoring" and support by increasing the adherence and the longevity of the application. Anchors are also very helpful close to joints. When the application is crossing a joint, which has a big range of motion and adds more strain on the tape during movement, anchors are always a good idea.

> Important: Anchors are *always* applied with absolutely no stretch!

## Duration of Application

A common question: "How long should these colorful strips stay on my dog?"

In most cases I recommend that when the tape doesn't fall off by itself and the dog doesn't start chewing on it, then the tape should be removed manually after three to four days. (Reminder: Always pull off the tape in the direction of the hair growth!)

Kinesiology tape has to endure a lot more when applied to a dog. The hair is the primary issue, but wind, rain, mud, and everyday dog activities can

*This combined Muscle-Tendon Taping for the biceps muscle/tendon is secured with three stretch-free crosswise anchors.*

cause the tape to come off. Many times, the applications will not last as long as they do on a human patient. Some tapings last a few days, others a week, and on rare occasions, there is an application that is made to last forever. That is when I get a phone call from a dog owner after 14 days or more asking me if the tape can now be removed from the dog. But that is the rare exception.

It is important to monitor your dog while he is taped and look for any signs of discomfort. When this occurs, you should remove the tape.

The most significant impact of a taping application happens within the first 24 hours. After that, the effect becomes less noticeable. Several days later, the body doesn't even "recognize" the tape stimulus anymore, so the response of the receptors in the tissue decreases. Most people who have been taped report that after three to four days they aren't aware of the tape anymore; this is when you can remove it. The same is advisable when taping dogs.

## Combination with Other Treatments

You can and should combine kinesiology taping with other treatment methods, since the tape was developed to be a supportive modality to other treatments. Massage, lymphatic drainage, acupuncture, stretching exercises, and manual therapy should be done before applying the tape. You can work with a magnetic blanket, laser therapy,

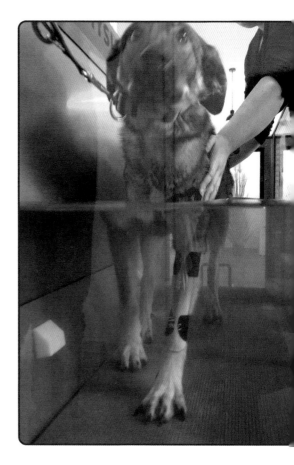

*Taping applications can be combined with other treatment modalities. Even a session in the water treadmill is possible with the tape.*

electro therapy, or ultrasound after the tape application. Once the tape is applied and adhering well to the hair, it can even get wet and dogs can use a water treadmill. But be careful when drying off the dog; don't rub over the tape with a towel—just gently dab it dry.

*This dog was Muscle Taped prior to doing pole exercises to activate and support the back muscles.*

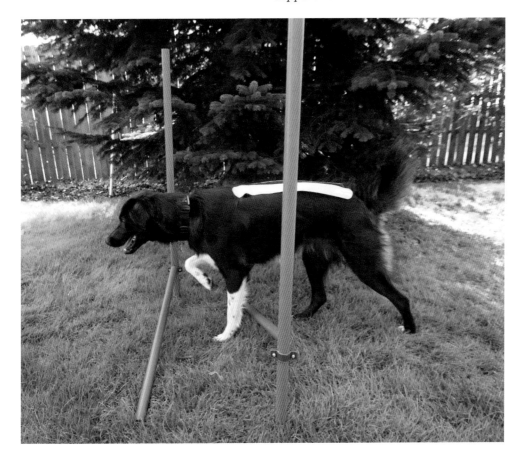

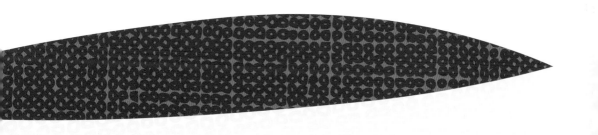

# Chapter 4:
# Before Getting Started

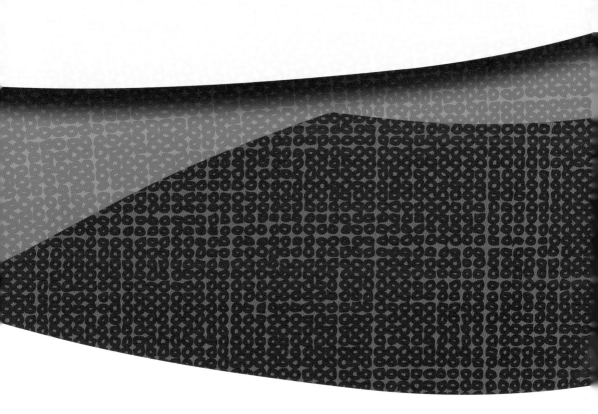

In this chapter, I explain and describe the many different taping applications, which, over time, have proven to be the most effective and are used most often. There are, of course, other taping applications, and every tape company and training institute has its own specific methods. There is also no limit to your own creativity, but you should always consider the following questions:

*While the dog owner is holding the extremity in the right position, the practitioner is applying a Proprioception Taping on the hind leg.*

- What are the dog's problems?

- How can these issues be helped with kinesiology tape?

- Does the hair length and body structure allow for a useful taping application?

- What do I want to achieve with the application? What is my goal?

- Which anatomical structure am I working on—muscle, fascia, tendon, ligament, bone, joint?

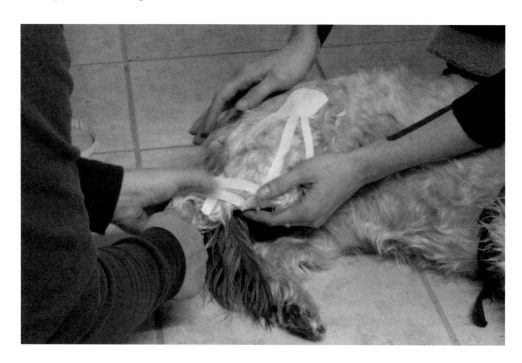

- Where exactly is this structure or body part? Where is the beginning and the end? What is important to consider around it?

Again and again, I see pictures of taped animals where I am left wondering what the practitioner was aiming for (often the tape is not following any

> A requirement for a reliable and successful taping application is a thorough and correct clinical examination. Kinesiology taping is a supportive treatment modality and is most effective in conjunction with veterinary, physiotherapy, osteopathy, and/or chiropractic treatment. Kinesiology taping is not a replacement for veterinary treatment.

kind of anatomical structure). Even after some consideration, the pictures and applications don't make sense to me. The effectiveness of kinesiology taping is still under scrutiny and there is hardly any scientific research or proof for it. This does not mean you should go out and start taping because it is nice and colorful, and looks pretty. In case of doubt, before using the tape, contact a veterinarian or animal physiotherapist with more taping experience to help you out. An experienced animal practitioner can explain the situation and problems to you, and recommend the right taping application, which should be the best to help your dog's current issue. Even I get regular calls and questions from fellow physiotherapists with little or no taping experience, asking me for help and advice—which I am always happy to give.

# Anatomical Terms

In the following section, I have tried to discuss taping applications in a general and easy-to-understand way and not use too many specific technical and anatomical terms. But sometimes you can't avoid it, especially when explaining the directions on a dog. For better understanding, you can find the most important terms here:

# Positional and Directional Terms for the Dog

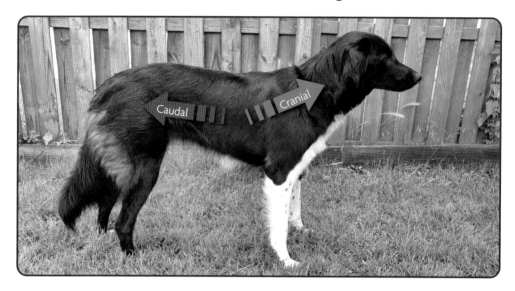

*Cranial: forward, toward the head. Caudal: backward, toward the tail.*

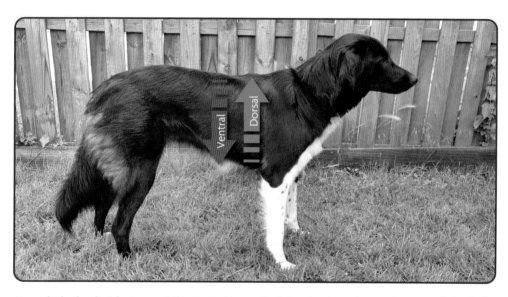

*Dorsal: the back side, toward the back. Ventral: abdominal, underneath, toward the belly.*

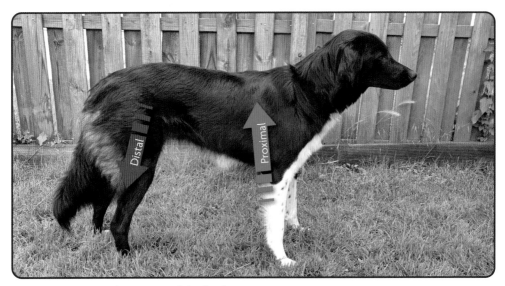

*Proximal: nearer the center of the body, toward the body. Distal: away from the center of the body, away from the body, toward the paw.*

## Terminology for Muscles

**Origin:** The attachment site of the muscle, which is proximal, closer to the body, and which does not move when the muscle contracts.

**Insertion:** The attachment site of the muscle, which is distal, farther away from the body, and moves when the muscle contracts.

**Hypertonic:** Higher muscle tone, increased muscle tension.

**Hypotonic:** Reduced muscle tone, less muscle tension.

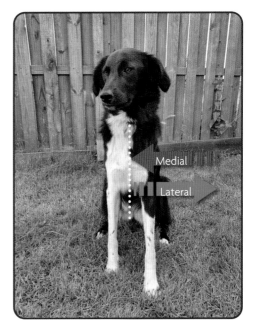

*Lateral: on the side, toward the side.*
*Medial: in the middle, toward the middle.*

**Hypertrophic:** Increased, enlarged muscle volume.

**Atrophic:** Decreased, reduced, under-developed muscle volume.

**Myogelosis or trigger point:** Area or point of palpable, tight, painful, chronic, and constant contraction in the muscle.

**Spasms:** Sudden, involuntary muscle cramps and contractions.

# Taping Terms

While handling kinesiology tape, there are also some specific terms that you will read about again and again, so here I will take a closer look at them and explain them in more detail.

## Backup

The *backup* is better described as a "push-back." When taping, you should always be using a backup when you lay down the stretch-free tape endings on the hair. This rule applies at the beginning of the tape strip as well as the end of the tape strip.

For example, when applying a single strip of kinesiology tape, running parallel with the hair growth (using the *End-to-End* technique), you apply the beginning of this tape strip (the primary end) with no stretch, and at the same time gently push this piece of tape back against the direction of the hair (backup) by using the flat palm of your

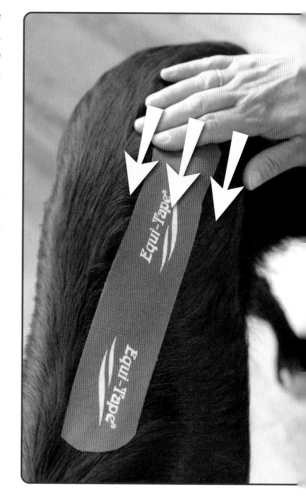

hand or flat fingers. This is an additional enhancement to the stretch- and tension-free beginning of the application.

The same is done at the end of the tape strip. The effective area of the tape is applied with the desired amount of stretch and the last 1 to 2 inches are applied stretch-free. Release any tension from this final piece of tape (secondary end) and push it back gently against the direction of the hair (backup).

Another example: When applying kinesiology tape that is stretched from the center outward (*Inside-Out* technique), like a *Decompression Tape*, the ends of the tape are also placed with no stretch. But, in this application, the direction of the backup is toward the center of the tape.

## Recoil

The technical definition for *recoil* is to rebound or spring back through the force of impact or elasticity. In

*The backup in the direction of the yellow arrows guarantees that the end of the tape strip will be stretch-free. Stretch and tension at the end of a tape strip can lead to an untimely detachment of the application.*

kinesiology taping, the best description would be to rebound through the force of elasticity.

Throughout this book, kinesiology tape has been described as stretchable; applications have a specific amount of stretch when placed onto a patient. Everything that is stretched has the desire to go back to its original un-stretched form (neutral-shape position). The tension that pulls the fibers of the kinesiology tape together to this neutral position is called *recoil*. With every taping application, keep this recoil effect in mind because you should consider what you want to achieve and, therefore, in which direction to tape and in which direction to point the recoil.

With the *End-to-End* technique, the tape recoils toward the primary end. When using the *Inside-Out* technique, it recoils toward the center of the tape. The direction of the recoil is always *opposite* the direction of the taping application.

Recoil has been described in detail, beginning on page 45 (about the basic taping technique), and you can also find more about it in the next chapter. It is demonstrated in the picture on page 72 on a *Muscle Taping* application.

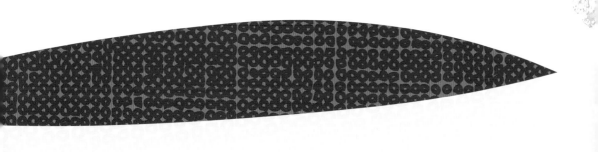

# Chapter 5:
# Various Taping
# Applications

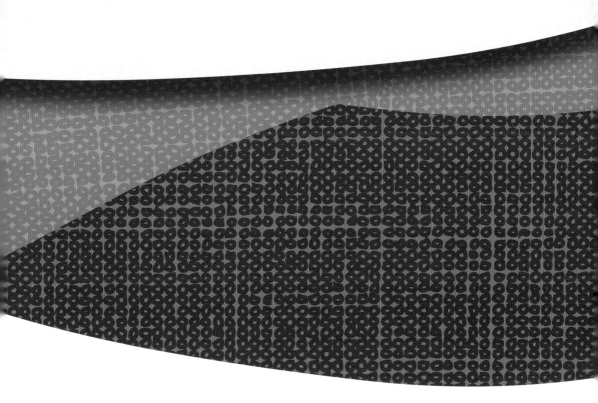

# Muscle Taping

There are three different types of muscles:

- **The smooth musculature:** These muscles are regulated by the Autonomic Nervous System (ANS), which unconsciously regulates the gut, heart, lungs, and other internal organs.

- **The cardiac musculature:** This is regulated by its very own heart sinus node, and it can only be found in the heart muscle, as indicated by the name. The cardiac muscle also cannot be controlled consciously.

- **The skeletal musculature:** These muscles are responsible for the movement of the body. They are attached via tendons to the skeleton and cross over bones and joints, and sometimes over two joints. During muscle contractions, the muscle fibers shorten, moving the attached bones closer to each other, while flexing the joint. When the muscles relax and stretch the muscle, fibers elongate and the bones move away from each other, causing the joint to straighten again. The skeletal musculature can be controlled voluntarily and cause the muscles to contract and relax.

Skeletal muscles are the ones you can and want to influence with kinesiology tape. Every muscle has a tendon of origin, a muscle belly with muscle fibers and a tendon of insertion. The tendons attach the muscle to the bone and the muscle belly goes over the articulated bone and joint.

The muscle belly consists of many muscle fibers and these fibers are made of millions of tiny muscle myofibrils. When the muscles contract, these tiny fibrils and filaments glide by each other and into each other. As a result, the muscle shortens, bringing the two bones closer to each other and movement begins. This is a very simplified version of muscle work, but it is the basic principle for muscle activity and the formation of motion. A requirement for an effective *Muscle Taping* is good anatomical knowledge of the skeletal musculature, the origin and insertion, and the direction of the muscle. The origin is usually closer to the body and attached to the less mobile bone. The insertion is usually farther away from the body and attached to the more mobile bone.

For example, let's look at the *M. longissimus*, the long back muscle. Anatomically this muscle consists of various segments: the *M. longissimus lumborum* (lumbar segment), the *M. longissimus thoracis* (thoracic segment), the *M. longissimus cervicis* (neck segment), and the *M. longissimus capitis* (head segment). But these segments all run parallel to the spine, transitioning smoothly into each other, one behind the other. The transitions of the segments are very fluid, and it is difficult to precisely separate one segment from the other. Since these transitions are so smooth it is generally referred to as one long muscle with its origin on the pelvis and sacrum, and the insertion is at the occiput, at the back of the head. When this muscle contracts and all four paws are solidly on the ground, the dog's back will hollow slightly. When the dog's front paws are off the ground, this muscle contraction supports him standing up on his hind legs, and when this muscle just contracts on one side of the spine, it is responsible for the lateral flexion of the body to the right or left.

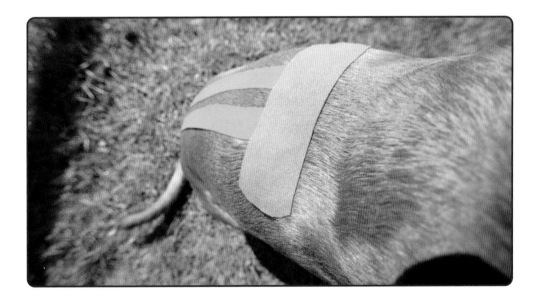

*The complete application of Muscle Taping on the M. longissimus with an additional stretch-free anchor crosswise at the primary end near the shoulder blades.*

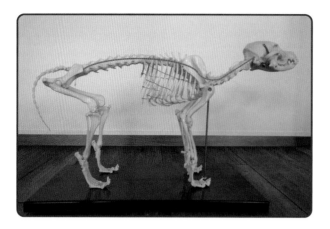

*The M. longissimus dorsi, the long back muscle (here schematically painted in a red line parallel to the spine) consists of multiple segments. The most frequent problems that can be treated with kinesiology tape are located in the lumbar and thoracic segments.*

If muscles are overworked, sore, tight, or maybe underdeveloped, you can help them with kinesiology tape in conjunction with massage, stretching, or manual therapy, for example.

## Application of a Muscle Taping

When taping a muscle, the muscle should be pre-stretched as much as possible. In the case of the long back muscle, the dog should be in the "sit" position and the dog's nose should point down toward the sternum if the dog can.

With other muscles, you should also try to position the dog so the muscle is stretched as much as the dog will allow. If you are trying to tape the larger muscles on the hind legs like the *M. semitendinosus, M. semimembranosus* or the *M. biceps femoris*, the dog should be lying on the side that isn't being treated while the leg to be taped is stretched cranially as much as possible without making the dog uncomfortable.

It is always helpful to have an assistant or dog owner to lend a hand when applying a *Muscle Taping*. The helper can encourage the dog to stay in the desired position until the tape has been fully applied.

In this pre-stretched position, the needed length of tape will be measured. In the case of the long back muscle, you can see in the picture on page 69 how the tape is measured from the top of the shoulder blade, parallel to the spine, to the highest point of the pelvis. While cutting the premeasured tape into shape and rounding the corners, the dog can remain in a more comfortable position.

After cutting the tape (if the dog is quite small and/or thin, it is a good idea to split the tape lengthwise), the dog should go back to the same sitting position as before, so that the back muscle remains pre-stretched until the tape strip is fully applied. For *Muscle Tapings*, you always use the *End-to-End* technique.

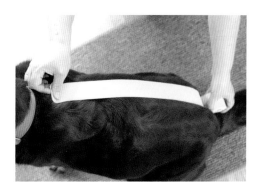

*After the clinical examination, the tape strip will be measured. The active area of the tape strip should cover the muscle belly completely—in this case, the M. longissimus.*

- About an inch (2 cm) from one end of the I-Tape, tear the paper backing completely across and remove the paper.

- This end (primary end) will be applied with absolutely no stretch at the insertion of the thoracic segment of the *M. longissimus* at the top of the shoulder blade. Push it back slightly with a backup.

- Remove the whole paper backing until the last inch (2 cm) of the tape strip.

- Be careful not to touch the now open adhesive layer with your fingers and don't let it make contact with the hair yet.

- Hold the end of the tape strip (secondary end) with flat fingers and with a little stretch (about 10 percent off-paper stretch) line it up along the direction of the muscle toward the sacrum, and with your other hand flat, apply the tape.

- Remove the paper backing from the last inch (2 cm) of the tape strip and apply this end (secondary end) with absolutely no stretch and a backup toward the muscle belly.

- Rub carefully but vigorously back and forth over the tape strip to create frictional heat and to activate the adhesive. After the application, let the dog stand up, lie down, or walk around.

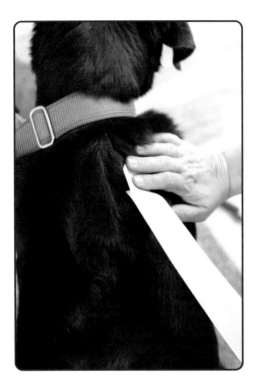

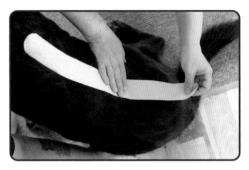

*The tape is applied with a mild stretch (about 10 to 20 percent stretch) along the affected area of the muscle.*

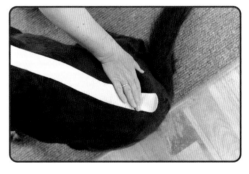

*The stretch-free primary end is positioned laterally to the spine and the tape strip is applied along the direction of the muscle.*

When the muscle returns to its normal position, like standing straight, after the kinesiology tape has been applied, you can oftentimes see that there are waves in the tape strip. These waves are called "convolutions" and they are absolutely normal. In addition, these waves increase the lifting effect.

*After applying the tape strip to the affected area, remove the paper backing from the secondary end, and put this end on stretch-free and with a "backup." In this case, the long back muscle has been taped from the insertion of the thoracic segment to the origin of the lumbar segment.*

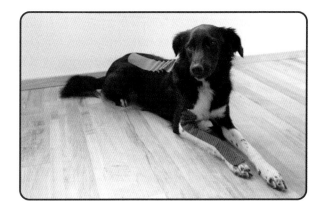

*Convolutions are an additional enhancement for the lifting effect. The purple Muscle Taping of the M. longissimus shows these waves very nicely.*

## Muscle Taping for the Long Back Muscle (M. longissimus)

**Direction of the tape:** Insertion to origin.

**Recoil:** Origin to insertion.

**Effect:** Support for the relaxation and stretching of the long back muscle.

## Activation or Relaxation of the Musculature?

Due to the aforementioned structure of the muscle, with its origin and insertion and its ability to contract, there are two possibilities for a *Muscle Taping* application: Activation and support of the muscle contraction or relaxation and stretching of the muscle.

When the muscle is working and contracting, the muscle fibers shorten and the mobile and more distal part is brought closer to the less mobile and more proximal part. In the case of the *M. longissimus*, the more mobile forehand is brought closer to the less mobile hindquarters.

When the muscle relaxes and the fibers elongate again, the insertion moves away from the origin. The mobile part (forehand) moves away from the immobile part (hindquarters) and the muscle stretches again.

Since kinesiology tape always recoils toward the primary end this leaves only two possibilities for the direction of the *Muscle Taping*:

**Activation** of the muscle (blue tape):

- Direction of the tape strip (black arrow): the primary end is located at the origin of the muscle, and the final end is located at the insertion of the muscle.

- Recoil (red arrow): toward the primary end at the origin of the muscle and along the direction of the muscle contraction.

**Relaxation** of the muscle (yellow tape):

- Direction of the tape strip (black arrow): The primary end is located at the insertion of the muscle and the secondary end is located at the origin of the muscle.

*The recoil of the tape strip is always opposite the direction of the taping application. The blue strip was taped caudally to cranially and the recoil goes to the primary caudal end. The yellow strip was taped cranially to caudally and the recoil again is going toward the primary end, which in this case is located cranially.*

- Recoil (red arrow): toward the primary end at the insertion of the muscle and along the direction of the muscle stretching.

Even with light or medium tension in the muscles, it is better to use the activation method, because you still want to support the muscle with the tape and improve muscle activity. When the muscle is absolutely tight and hard as a rock, it is time to use the relaxation method.

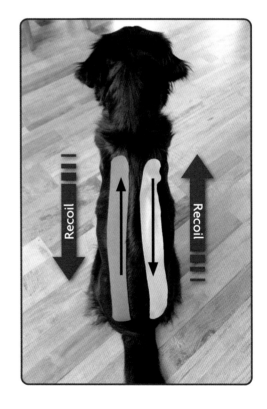

### Unilateral or Bilateral Muscle Taping

I am a big advocate of bilateral muscle taping. This means that even if the problem is only on one side—for example, a tight back muscle on the left side—I will also tape the right side of the back muscle in the same manner as the left.

In my experience, animals do not process the stimulation as logically as we humans do, and they react primarily to the stimulus of the tape. A unilateral taping application can lead to issues of crookedness in the posture and maybe an uneven gait. For example, with horses in training, you can see the change, and riders can feel it when on the horse. This distortion is also not desirable when taping dogs, especially since it is more challenging to recognize since we don't ride them. Our goal in each treatment should be to improve the biomechanics of the animal, not to make the dog even more crooked because the muscle is only being taped on one side.

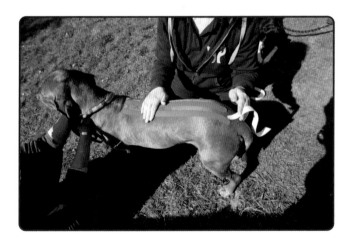

*Bilateral taping application for the long back muscle. Both tape strips have the same direction of taping and the same amount of stretch. They run parallel on the right and left sides of the spine.*

### Caution

When a muscle is taped bilaterally and one of the tape strips starts to detach itself, always remove both tape strips at the same time to avoid a crooked posture or an uneven gait.

# Lymphatic Taping

## Lymphatic Fluid and Lymphatic System

*Lympha* is actually an ancient Greek word that was later transferred to Latin and means "clear water." And that is what lymphatic fluid really looks like: a clear, yellowish fluid that is the intermediate stage between blood plasma and tissue fluid. Delicate lymphatic capillaries absorb the free lymphatic fluid within the tissue. These capillaries join into larger lymphatic vessels and these empty into the lymphatic nodes, which are a collection point and filter for the lymphatic

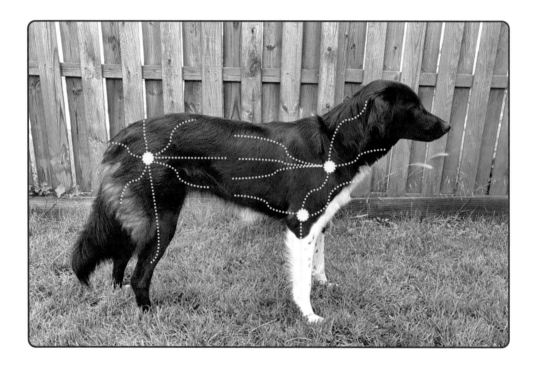

*Schematic drawing of the most important lymph node centers and their areas of inflow. With the help of Lymphatic Taping the reabsorption and backflow of fluid buildup to these nodes will be supported.*

fluid. From these nodes, the lymphatic fluid is transported to the subclavian veins where it is reabsorbed into the bloodstream. In the picture you can see a schematic drawing of the most important lymph node areas: the axillary lymph node on the inside of the front leg and the inguinal lymph node on the inside of the hind leg as well as the main lymphatic node at the subclavian vein just in front of the shoulder blade. The lines indicate the direction of inflow for each lymphatic node.

The lymphatic fluid carries substances that can't be transported in the bloodstream. The lymph nodes not only clean and filter the lymphatic fluid but also contain *lymphocytes*. Lymphocytes are an important part of the immune system, defending the body against disease by fighting against antibodies that don't belong in the system.

Through infection, injury, and sometimes even an operation, lymphatic fluid builds up in dogs' extremities. Due to increased volume and enlarged pressure on the delicate lymphatic capillaries, these are squeezed shut and no longer able to reabsorb free fluid and move it to the lymph nodes.

In these situations, a lymphatic drainage is most helpful: a special, very gentle form of massage, which stimulates the lymphatic system and the main nodes to improve the fluid movement. To further support the manual lymphatic drainage, a *Lymphatic Taping* can be applied on the affected extremity.

## The Application of a Lymphatic Taping

The most important tape cut for this application is the Fan-Tape, which can be combined to create a lymphatic row or a lymphatic grid, depending on the size and shape of the swelling. The Fan-Tape has one closed end (primary end) and three to five fingers (see p. 44). The more fingers you cut for the Fan-Tape, the more surface you can cover by spreading the fingers out.

The *End-to-End* technique is used for the Fan-Tape and you always apply the closed primary end first and then one fan finger at a time.

After cutting the Fan-Tape into shape, tear the paper backing between the primary end and where the fingers begin and fold the paper backing over a little. This will help you grab hold of the fingers and the paper backing more easily and quickly when applying the tape.

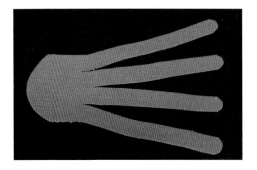

*For the Lymphatic Taping, the Fan-Tape is used, with its one closed end and its multiple "fingers" at the other end.*

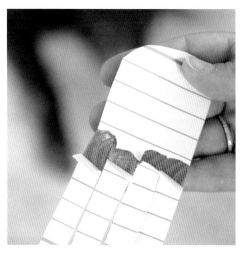

## General Application of Lymphatic Tape

- Remove the paper backing completely from the closed end.

- Apply the end of the Fan-Tape at the lymphatic node pointing proximally and with absolutely no stretch.

- Take the torn paper backing of the first finger and point it distally toward the swelling.

- Since the tape comes off the paper backing with 10 percent pre-stretch, you don't need to add more than a mild stretch when the finger is applied in the distal direction toward the swelling. Or just use the off-paper stretch.

*To better apply the tape and get a good hold of the paper backing, tear it at the spot between the primary end and the fingers, and fold the paper over a bit as shown.*

- The end of this finger will again be applied with absolutely no stretch.

- Use the same procedure with all the other fingers as well and spread them out generously over the swelling.

- The tape fingers can, thereby, be applied in a straight line or in a wave line. The wave lines enable you to cover even more surface.

- If it is a large swelling on the front or hind legs, it is helpful to start applying the two outside fingers first and kind of framing the swelling on the right and left sides. Then you can apply and spread the middle fingers evenly over the swollen area.

- When rubbing over the tape to activate the adhesive, it is better to start from the primary end and work toward the end of the fingers. If you start at the fingers, you risk detaching the thin finger ends by accident.

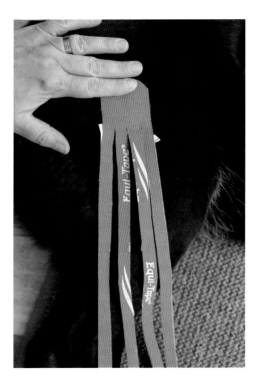

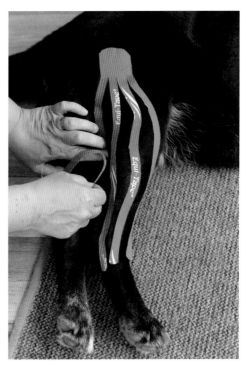

*Remove the paper backing at the primary end. Point this end toward the closest lymphatic node and apply it with no stretch.*

*The fingers of the lymphatic tape are applied with a mild stretch (about 10 percent as it comes off the paper backing) around and over the swelling in the direction of the paw.*

## The Lymphatic Row

The "lymphatic row" is suitable for larger dogs, and depending on their size you can apply two or three Fan-Tapes in a row. For smaller dogs, one Fan-Tape is usually enough. The lymphatic row is used when the swelling affects the whole extremity.

When applying a lymphatic row on the front legs, start at the primary lymph node at the subclavian vein just in front of the shoulder blade (bend the head and neck slightly toward the opposite side) and work the fingers down toward the paw. Like a traffic jam, you have to clear the congestion at the beginning (lymph node), and you have to make space for the "cars" (the lymphatic fluid) to "drive on" (flow out).

When taping larger dogs with two or more Fan-Tapes in a row, it is important that the end of the next Fan-Tape is applied overlapping the finger endings of the previous Fan-Tape. You want to create a "lymphatic row" and a continuous lymphatic backflow throughout

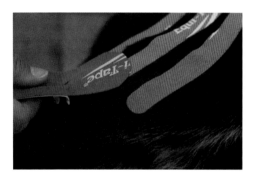

*Important for the lymphatic row: the end of the following (lower) Fan-Tape is applied on top of the finger endings of the previous Fan-Tape to ensure that the lymphatic row is continuous and there is no gap in between.*

*When there is a larger swelling, covering the whole extremity, multiple Fan-Tapes can be applied in a lymphatic row.*

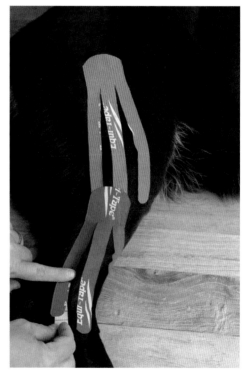

the whole extremity toward the lymphatic node.

## The Lymphatic Grid

When there are swollen areas within the extremity—for example, around the carpal joint of the front leg or the tarsal joint of the hind leg—the lymphatic grid is primarily used. Instead of building a row, you take two or more Fan-Tapes and apply them at the same height. The ends are all pointed proximally toward the lymphatic node but are shifted against each other at an angle. The fingers of the different Fan-Tapes are applied crosswise over the swelling and pointing distally so that it results in a grid-like pattern. This grid should encircle and cover the swelling as much as possible.

You can also combine a lymphatic row with a lymphatic grid. Start proximally with the row and then add several Fan-Tapes as a grid around a swollen joint.

This always depends on the individual situation, swelling, and also the size of the dog. The extremity of a Jack Russell Terrier is so short that you can cover a whole leg with just one Fan-Tape. For a Doberman Pinscher, you might need two to three Fan-Tapes.

I recommended securing all the thin and delicate finger endings of a *Lymphatic Tape* with an anchor (this anchor can be seen in light blue in the picture on p. 80). Anchors

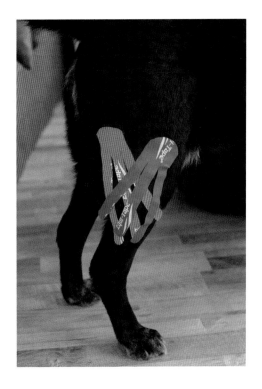

*For larger swellings on an extremity, you can apply several Fan-Tapes next to each other, so that they are building a grid-like pattern. The ends of the Fan-Tapes are still pointed proximally toward the lymphatic node, just at different angles.*

are single I-Tapes that are applied around the extremity and over the finger endings without any stretch, to cover, secure, and protect the finger endings of the Fan-Tape without compromising or restricting the actual taping application. It is, therefore, very important to always apply these anchors without any stretch at all (see p. 49)!

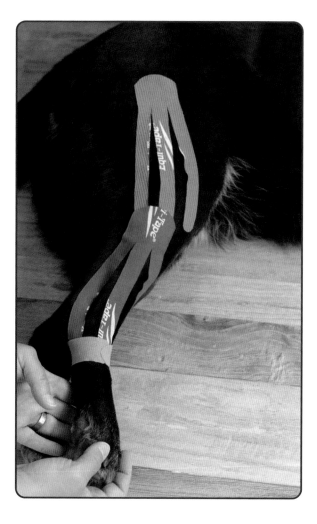

*To secure the taping application and especially all the thin and delicate finger endings, you should cover and protect them with a stretch-free anchor.*

## Lymphatic Taping
**Direction of tape:** from the lymphatic node toward the swelling.
**Recoil:** from the swelling toward the lymphatic node.
**Effect:** supporting the backflow of fluid buildup in the extremities toward the lymph node.

# Scar Taping

## Scar Tissue

Scar tissue is formed as a wound heals after an injury or surgical incisions in the deeper layers of the skin. Injuries such as burns or cuts are the most common. Unfortunately, the body is not capable of rebuilding the damaged body structures exactly as they were before. Soft tissue is replaced by fibrous connective tissue. Normally these fibers are part of the healthy connective tissue and are generally arranged in a parallel order. Unfortunately, with scar tissue, the fibers are irregular, and grow crisscrossed and uncontrolled and disorganized into the existing tissue. This can lead to areas where hair roots, sebaceous glands, and sweat glands are destroyed and cannot be rebuilt. Therefore, regular skin function in these areas can be damaged—if not destroyed.

Excessive growth of fibrous scar tissue can lead to scar proliferations or scar bulging. When there is too little growth of the fibrous connective tissue, the scar often looks sunken in or retracted. This can be seen with muscle fiber injuries, which leave an indentation in the muscle belly. These are scars in the deeper layers of the muscle.

The important point is that because of these fibers, this connective tissue is mostly less elastic than the skin and tissue it replaces. If a scar is located near a joint or on a structure close to a joint that is used mechanically, it can lead to a restriction in the range of motion. Scar tissue can also block the energy flow in the body if it crosses and interferes with the course of one or more meridians.

The aim of a scar-tissue treatment/ massage is to soften the tissue and increase the elasticity as well as the energy flow. As a support to this treatment, a *Scar Taping* is always very helpful.

A scar treatment and applying a *Scar Taping* should only be done once a wound has completely healed from the outside. This means:
- When the wound is fully closed on the outside.
- When the scab has fallen off by itself.
- When all surgical sutures have been removed by a veterinarian.

The newer a scar is, the greater the chances for successful treatment. But even scars that are a few years old can still be treated effectively. Most of the time, it will take a lot longer because the replaced connective tissue can get more and more rigid and inelastic over time.

Scar treatments and *Scar Taping* are usually not a one-time thing. This tissue can be really "stiff and stubborn" and, therefore, requires multiple treatments. In some cases, this can take several months, during which the scar needs weekly treatment, massage, and taping.

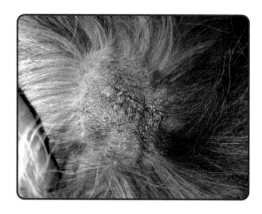

*A fresh scar after the removal of a tumor. When the stitches have been removed, the Scar Taping can be applied.*

## The Application of a *Scar Taping*

Depending on the size and length of the scar, many little strips of tape will be needed. Unlike the large strips, the corners of these little strips don't need to be rounded. But pay attention! They still need to be cut lengthwise and not vertically, since they are not stretchable in that direction. With *Scar Taping*, the *Inside-Out* technique will be used.

• Take the first little tape strip, tear the paper backing in the middle and remove the paper on both sides just before the end.

• Give the tape a medium stretch and apply it at a 45-degree angle to the scar. The center of the I-Tape is directly on top of the scar.

• Apply both ends of the little I-strip with no stretch.

• The second little tape strip is applied at a 45-degree angle to the scar in the opposite direction. So it turns out like a little cross—an X.

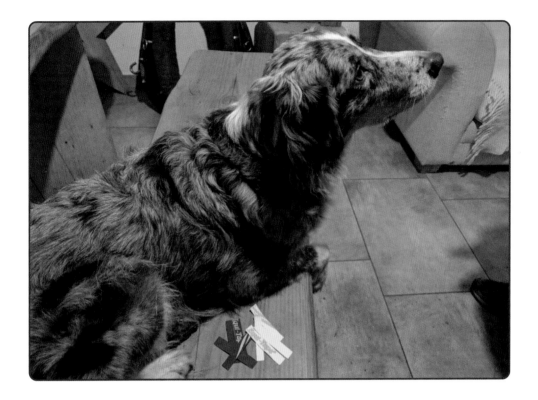

*For a Scar Taping, several little tape strips are needed. As an exception to the rule, these don't have to be cut with rounded corners.*

- This second little tape strip is applied in the same manner as the first: tear the paper in the middle and remove it just until the ends, center it over the scar, and apply with medium stretch, using the *Inside-Out* technique with no stretch in the ends.

- Repeat this alternating application as you work your way along the scar. The third strip is applied parallel to

the first one, and the fourth one parallel to the second, and so on.

- Each cross (X) is applied next to another, going all along the length of the scar so that at the end, the application looks like a lattice fence.

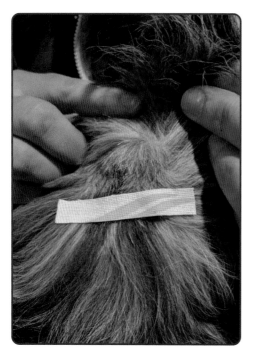 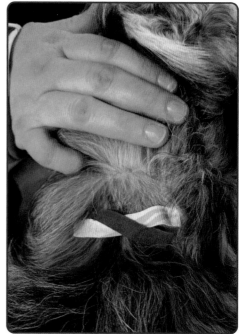

*The stitches have been removed and the hair has grown in a little bit. The first tape strip is applied with the Inside-Out technique and medium stretch at a 45-degree angle to the scar.*

*The second tape strip is also applied using the Inside-Out technique but this strip is placed at a 45-degree angle in the opposite direction of the first one, so that the two strips create an X.*

### Tip

Because of the two different colors of tape strips, the Xs can be seen more clearly. This is also helpful in everyday practice. When you have a more extensive scar, you can accidentally lose the direction of taping and inadvertently continue with the direction of the first tape or, in this case, the blue tape strips. When using two colors, you can immediately notice and see where the pattern of the X (the "lattice fence") is incorrect.

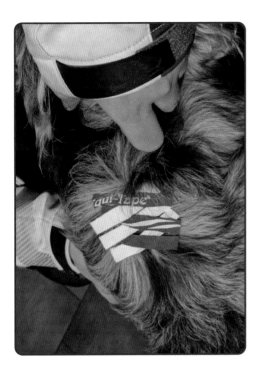

*With this X pattern you work your way along the length of the scar until it is completely covered from one end to the other. In the end, the application looks like a lattice fence. It is okay to leave little gaps between the tape strips.*

- When the whole scar is covered with a "lattice fence," you cut one or more regular-sized I-Tapes with rounded corners, depending on the size of the *Scar Taping.*

- These I-Tapes are also applied with the *Inside-Out* Technique, tearing the paper in the middle and using very little stretch. But they are applied parallel to the actual scar above the "lattice fence" to cover and protect it.

- The ends are applied with no stretch, as always.

- Depending on the size of the scar and the size of the dog, the bigger I-Tapes sometimes just cover the right and left side of the "lattice fence," and sometimes they cover the entire application.

- Afterward, carefully rub over the whole taping application to create frictional heat and to activate the adhesive.

The bigger I-Tapes are not only an anchor and protection for the "lattice fence" underneath it. Since the small overlapping strips are applied with medium stretch and the big I-Tapes are applied with light stretch, an interaction between the layers of tape is created. This gives the actual scar tissue additional stimulation—first, through the directly applied grid, and second, through the interaction of the layers of tape.

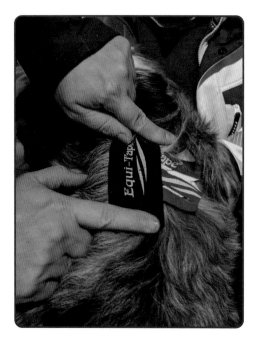
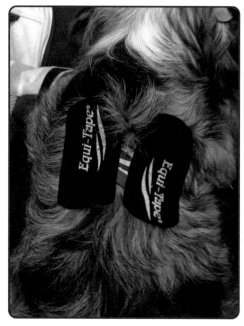

*To secure the application and give an additional parallel taping impulse to the scar tissue, it is covered with a lightly stretched cross-anchor (Inside-Out technique).*

*For larger Scar Tapings, several cross-anchors can be used. The outside borders of the "lattice fence" underneath should be totally covered.*

In addition, there will be another impulse from a different direction for the scar tissue through this top taping layer. The bottom layer stimulates the scar from two different diagonal directions, and the top layer stimulates the tissue from a parallel direction.

Scar Taping
**Direction of the tape:** multiple directions away from the scar.
**Recoil:** from multiple directions toward the scar.
**Effect:** support of the regeneration of inelastic, disturbed, and scarred connective tissue.

# Fascia Taping

Fascia is part of the connective tissue. In contrast to the aforementioned scar tissue, fascia is not rigid or inelastic. On the contrary: fasciae are wafer-thin layers of parallel-arranged connective tissue that encase muscles and muscle fibers, as well as inner organs. Fascia works as a protective layer and is crucial for the muscle's smooth contraction and stretching by letting the different fibers glide by each other. For years fascia was not considered to be an essential body tissue and has been largely neglected and overlooked.

However, treatment and massage of connective tissue isn't new and has been done for about 100 years. With today's research and studies, scientists now know how vital fascia and connective tissue are for the body. Over the years, special fascia techniques have been developed, but even with regular massage, the superficial fascia will be stimulated due to the fact that it encases the muscles being massaged. Since everything is connected through fascia chains, you can even reach deeper layers of tissue and fascia through special fascia techniques.

Nowadays, there is a substantial body of research on fascia tissue and scientists have found out that these wafer-thin structures play a major role in every aspect of the body. This layer of connective tissue contains a lot of sensory cells and nerve cells; it is instrumental to the body's proprioception and body awareness. Some scientists now even think of fascia as an organ and call it the most important organ of the body since it is everywhere and connects everything.

So what does fascia look like?

If you have ever cut a chicken breast, you have seen fascia without being aware of it. The chicken breast is often covered by a very thin and delicate whitish, milky "skin-like" layer. This is fascia! In the case of the chicken breast, the fascia layer (shown in the picture on p. 98) is really, really thin. But there are areas on larger animals and also humans where this layer can be much thicker and stronger, such as the lumbar region.

Fascia can thicken and stiffen in response to trauma, surgery, or through extreme or constant strain and overloading. This tightening compromises the shear motion of the fascia and the tissue. Muscle fibers cannot glide by each other smoothly when supposed to be contracting or relaxing, resulting in limited movement and pain. These small fascia changes have an impact on muscle activity as well as other parts of the body, such as inner organs, since they are covered by fascia as well.

These tied-up fascia structures can be worked on and released with massage and special fascia techniques. *Fascia Taping* is an excellent modality to support this work.

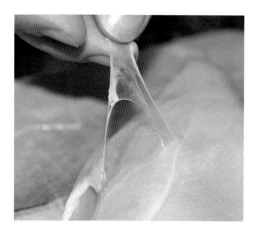

*Fascia is a thin delicate layer of connective tissue, covering muscles as well as inner organs. When cutting up a chicken breast it can be seen as thin, whitish, milky skin, covering the meat.*

## The Application of *Fascia Taping*

*Fascia Taping* applications aim to release tense or restricted fasciae, to reorganize the affected tissue, restore the original functional status, and give full range of motion. There are two *Fascia Taping* applications, and you can either use a single I-Tape, a Y-Tape, or a Fan-Tape for both. It all depends on the area and size of the compromised fascia tissue. For smaller areas and small dogs, an I-Tape might be sufficient. For larger areas or bigger dogs, a Fan-Tape is often the right choice since you can split up the fingers and, therefore, cover a larger surface.

No matter which tape cut is chosen, you will always use the *End-to-End* technique.

When palpating the afflicted area, the fascia can not only be tense but may feel like it is actually pulling you in one direction, or that one direction feels more mobile than the other.

This direction of mobility/immobility is key to determining the direction of the taping application and the recoil created. You want to loosen and relax the fascia and not work in the wrong direction with the tape's recoil, possibly worsening the situation.

Once you have palpated the fascia and found the direction where the fascia is free and mobile, your tape strip is applied in this "free" direction.

Since the tape always recoils toward the primary end, against the direction of the application, the fascia will get an impulse in the opposite direction: in the direction that is less mobile, or more tied up and tense. Through this recoil, you can enhance relaxation, mobility, and loosening up of the fascia.

### Variation 1—Alternating *Tape Stretch*

In this variation, the fascia is stimulated with different amounts of stretch within the tape strip.

- Tear the paper backing across about one inch (2 to 3 cm) from one end of the tape strip, and remove it completely.

- This primary end is applied with no stretch as usual, and can be supported with a backup.

- Remove the rest of the paper backing until about one inch (2 to 3 cm) before the other end, and give the tape strip a medium to strong stretch.

- Apply about one inch (2 to 3 cm) of the tape with this amount of stretch.

- Then release the stretch from the tape and hold it, so it is barely stretched and not dangling.

- Apply about an inch (2 to 3 cm) with barely any stretch.

- After that, apply another inch (2 to 3 cm) with the medium to strong stretch.

- And then another inch (2 to 3 cm) with barely any stretch.

- Keep on applying the alternating tape sections of stretch and no stretch until you reach the end of the tape strip.

- This secondary end is applied absolutely stretch-free and with a backup.

- Rub over the application carefully but vigorously to activate the adhesive through frictional heat.

If you have a small dog, the alternating sections of tape stretch/no stretch should, of course, be shorter; instead of one inch (2 to 3 cm) choose half an inch (about 1 cm). With this variation of *Fascia Taping,* the tissue gets multiple little impulses toward the direction of the strain to stimulate the reorganization and relaxation of the fascia.

While applying the kinesiology tape, make sure to hold the tape with flat fingers to avoid uneven stretch within the strip.

When applying a Y-Tape or a Fan-Tape with this variation, every single finger is applied with the variation mentioned above.

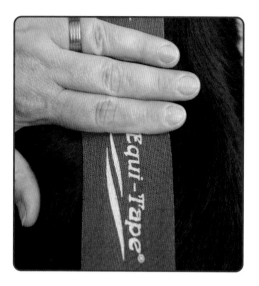

*Variation 1: This variation of a Fascia Taping uses sections of alternating amounts of stretch to help the tissue to reorganize and relax. A section with medium to strong stretch alternates with a section with barely any stretch. The logo on the tape is a great visual for the different amounts of stretch. When being stretched the logo appears distorted; without stretch, the logo looks normal.*

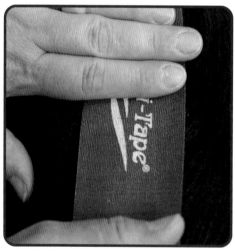

The kinetic energy of the vibration is transferred to the kinesiology tape and then transported farther into the fascia tissue. (Energy never gets lost! It just changes to another level and maybe another shape/form.)

The shape of the tape strip is chosen according to the size and area of the afflicted tissue.

- Remove the paper backing from the first inch (2 to 3 cm) of the tape strip.

- Apply the primary end with no stretch and support it with a backup.

- Remove the rest of the paper backing until the last 1 or 2 inches (3 to 4 cm) and give the tape a light stretch.

### Variation 2—Even Tape Stretch and Vibration

With the second variation, there is an even stretch in the tape strip. The fascia is stimulated manually with vibrations to relax and reorganize it.

- Your free hand is placed onto the tape just behind the primary end.

- Palpate through the tape strip into the fascia layer and start vibrating the fascia, thereby stimulating it.

- Work your way along the afflicted area, while applying the tape strip with light stretch and under constant vibration.

- The end (secondary end) is applied stretch-free as usual and with a backup and no vibration.

- Rub over the tape to activate the adhesive with frictional heat.

*When applying a Variation 2 Fascia Taping, the tape is stretched evenly and lightly. The free hand palpates through the material into the fascia and starts vibrating the fascia with a high frequency—here represented schematically with the yellow arrow.*

When using a Y-Tape or Fan-Tape, every finger is applied with the Variation 2 method mentioned above.

With this variation, one hand is busy with the guidance, direction, and light stretch of the tape. At the same time the other hand, using flat fingers, stimulates the fascia through vibration.

Both variations work very effectively, and it is usually a personal preference in the handling, as to which application to choose—Variation 1 or 2.

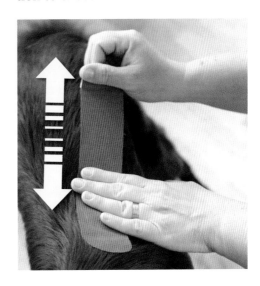

## Fascia Taping

**Direction of the tape:** in the direction where the fascia is free and mobile.

**Recoil:** in the direction where the fascia is afflicted and immobile.

**Effect:** support of mobilization of tight and/or tense fascia restrictions.

# Decompression Taping

Whenever a dog has a very localized problem, a *Decompression Taping* is recommended. Due to its form and effect, it is also known as *Star Tape*, *Space Tape*, *Pain Cross*, and sometimes it is lovingly called *Flower Tape*. It has a very strong localized effect, which is created by applying multiple tape strips on top of each other in the area of concern.

Through this overlay of tape strips, the lifting effect in the center of the application multiplies and a lot of space is created to decompress the tissue, reducing pain.

**Trigger Points**
Trigger points are localized, very tight spots within a muscle. Those points can be extremely painful and even cause pain in the surrounding body tissue.

**Misalignment and Blocking in Joints**
When resolving blockings/misalignments in joints, like in between vertebrae, the soft tissue surrounding the area is also affected. The tissue can be tight, restricted, and/or painful. Therefore, it is helpful to treat the soft tissue nearby to prevent repetitive misalignments.

**Arthrosis**
A lot of pain most often accompanies arthritis and arthrosis, like hip or elbow arthrosis. This side effect of pain can be reduced with the *Decompression Taping*, allowing the sore tissue to relax.

## The Application of a Decompression Taping

A *Decompression Taping* always consists of four equally long I-Tapes. The length depends on the size of the dog and the affected area. When taping smaller dogs, it is wise to split the tape in half lengthwise because the application might otherwise be too big for the dog. For *Decompression Taping*, the *Inside-Out* technique is always used.

- Tear the paper backing in the middle of the first tape strip and remove it on both sides until an inch before the ends.

- Hold the tape strip on both ends with flat fingers, center it over the affected area, and apply it with a medium to strong stretch horizontally.

- Remove the paper backing from the ends one at a time, and without any stretch, apply and backup.

- Rub over the tape carefully but vigorously to activate the adhesive through frictional heat.

- Take the second tape strip, and tear the paper backing in the middle, and remove paper until one inch before the ends.

- Place the second strip at a right angle to the first one, center it, and apply with a little less stretch than the first one. Then apply both ends stretch-free.

- Don't forget to rub over the second strip to activate the adhesive.

- Continue with the third and fourth strips in the same manner but place them diagonal to the first strip, one tilted to the left and one tilted to the right. Each tape strip should have a little less stretch than the previous one.

- Rub over each diagonal tape strip separately to activate the adhesive.

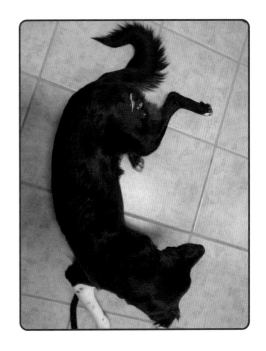

*A Decompression Taping after a bad spill and a bruised hip joint.*

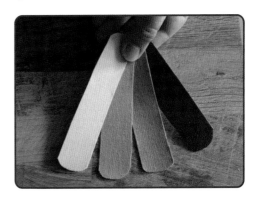

*For a Decompression Taping, you need four I-Tapes, which are equally long and wide.*

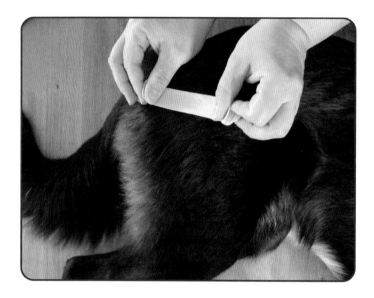

*The first tape strip of the Decompression Taping is applied with medium stretch and Inside-Out technique as horizontally as possible onto the affected area (in this case, the hip joint).*

It is essential to pay attention to the amount of stretch in each tape strip. From the first to the fourth strip, the amount of stretch should decrease. Otherwise, the last tape strip on the top might have so much stretch that it pulls on the other tape strips underneath. The whole application would then be under too much tension, which could cause a premature detachment of the entire application!

There are now four layers of tape over the affected area, applied with the *Inside-Out* technique. Each layer lifts the tissue a little bit, and therefore, the lifting effect increases and actually multiplies, creating a lot of space in the tight tissue area, and this body part will decompress.

## Decompression Taping

**Direction of the tape:** away and toward the outside of the affected area.

**Recoil:** toward the center of the affected area.

**Effect:** support of tissue decompression in a tight spot, creates lots of space locally.

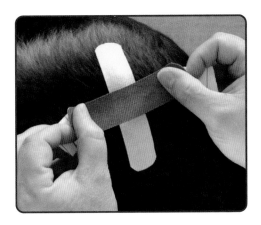

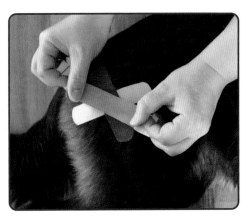

*The second tape strip is applied with light to medium stretch at a right angle to the first strip. It results in a "+"-like shape.*

*The third strip of tape is applied with light stretch at a 45-degree angle between the first and the second strip.*

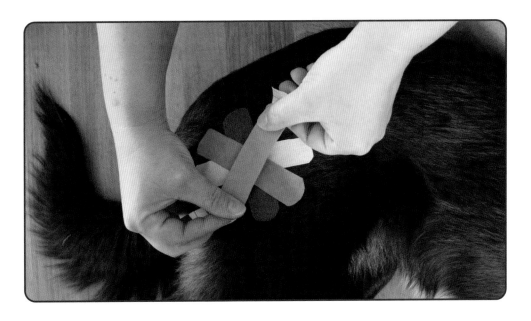

*The fourth and last I-Tape is applied with a minimum stretch in a right angle to the previous third tape strip. The completed application of the Decompression Taping looks a lot like a star, and that is why it is often referred to as a Star Tape.*

# Hematoma Taping

A hematoma is a bruised area where blood vessels burst and cause a blood-filled blister at the area of impact, usually under the skin. I think almost everyone has at least once in their life hit their elbow or shin, which resulted in a blueish bruise afterward. Dogs can also get hematomas—for example, after a bad spill or after a bite from another dog, and sometimes even after a poorly placed vaccine injection. Due to their hair coat, the discoloration is not visible and many times a hematoma can only be detected by a bump or swelling.

When the blood clots up at a localized spot, the tension in that area increases, causing pressure on the pain receptors. The outflow of waste products can be affected as well, and it can be really painful. A *Hematoma Taping* can bring relief in these cases.

## The Application of a Hematoma Taping

Similar to the *Lymphatic Taping,* the primary tape-cut is the Fan-Tape with one closed end and three to five fingers, which are applied using the *End-to-End* technique. As described in the *Lymphatic Taping* (see p. 75), once you have cut the tape fingers, the paper backing should be torn and folded at the transition from the end to each finger. This makes it easy to quickly grab hold of the paper when applying the Fan-Tape.

The length and number of Fan-Tapes depend on the size of the affected area and the hematoma. The larger the swelling, the more Fan-Tapes will be needed to create as much outflow as quickly as possible, easing the pressure on the tissue. The primary end is always placed outside the swelling while the fingers are pointed and applied toward the swelling. This creates a recoil away from the swelling, which supports the outflow of the fluid buildup.

- The primary end always points away from the hematoma/swelling.

- Remove the paper backing completely from the end and apply with no stretch.

- Apply tape fingers with a light (10 percent) stretch, just as they come off the paper backing.

- Grab the torn paper backing of one of the outer fingers and gently pull it off toward the hematoma. Apply the tape finger immediately with this off-paper stretch along the edge of the swelling.

- The end of the tape finger is applied with no stretch as usual.

- Put down the other outer finger in the same manner, along the other edge of the swelling, to encase the swelling as much as possible.

- The inner fingers are also applied in this manner but spread out evenly and directly over the swelling.

- The fingers can either be taped in straight lines or in a wavy pattern. The wave pattern lets you cover more surface area when the swelling is really big.

- All finger endings are put down without any stretch at all.

- When rubbing over the tape to activate the adhesive, make sure the motion is directed from the primary end to the fingers. In the other direction, you are at risk of accidentally rubbing off the finger endings of the kinesiology tape.

All other needed Fan-Tapes are applied the same way, but their ends

**Important Note**
In cases where the swelling is positioned directly above an extremity—for example, on the shoulder blade or near the hip—you should never apply a Fan-Tape with the end pointing distally toward the paw. Even though it is good to create as many directions for the outflow as possible, it is not wise to direct the fluid into an extremity. The fluid could build up in the leg, get stuck there, and then need to be transported away from there against the pull of gravity.

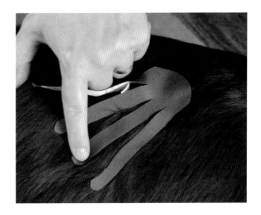

*For a Hematoma Taping, you will always use the Fan-Tape. It is applied so that the fingers cover and encase the hematoma completely. The primary end of the Fan-Tape is always placed outside of the swelling.*

should always point in different directions. This promotes and enhances the outflow of waste products in multiple directions: the more Fan-Tapes, the better the outflow.

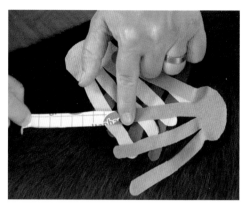

*Here the completed application has three directions of outflow. The first is pointed dorso-cranial, the second dorso-caudal, and the last one is pointed cranial. A fourth Fan-Tape could have been placed in addition, pointing caudally, opposite to the blue tape.*

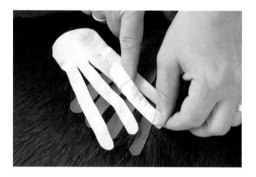

*Depending on the size of the swelling, multiple Fan-Tapes can be used. The tape fingers of the second Fan-Tape also cover and encase the swelling. The end also points away from the swelling but in a different direction to create a secondary outflow for the waste products and fluid buildup.*

## Hematoma Taping

**Direction of the tape**: toward the hematoma/swelling.

**Recoil**: away from the hematoma/ swelling.

**Effect**: supporting the outflow of stocked-up fluids in the area of the abdomen.

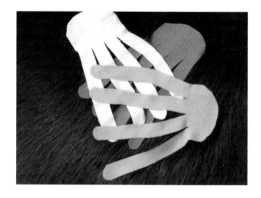

*There is a simple rule for Hematoma Tapings: the more, the better. The more Fan-Tapes, the more directions for the outflow!*

# Stabilization Taping

Some dogs have problems with the stability of their body, which is mostly a result of their anatomy, posture, or gait. As a result, you will often find tension in these areas as well as misalignments of the joints. Misalignments can be found between the vertebrae of the spine, as well as in the joints of the extremities such as shoulders, elbows, knees, and even the hips. Dogs with long backs, bow legs, or knock knees are just a few that suffer from stability issues. Another group is dogs with weak connective tissue and poor musculature, which have trouble building up and keeping up muscles. Puppies that are growing too fast or unevenly and are a little out of proportion can also have stability issues.

The body has many areas that are susceptible to weakness and misalignments. On the spine, the most commonly affected area for instability is the transition between the lumbar spine and sacrum as well as the sacroiliac joints. Another problem area is the transition between the base of the skull and the first and second vertebrae. The transition from the cervical spine to the thoracic spine can also be a problem.

A *Stabilization Taping* can bring stability to these areas and support the joints.

## The Application of a Stabilization Taping

Depending on the body region, a *Stabilization Taping* can vary quite drastically. For example, some areas like the spine are easier to reach with kinesiology tape than an elbow joint. Therefore, you can have multiple application variations for *Stabilization Taping*.

### Spine

For a *Stabilization Taping* of the spine, you need four I-Tapes. The length depends on the size of the dog. For smaller dogs, it is helpful to split the tape strips in half lengthwise. The *Inside-Out* technique will be used.

Similar to *Decompression Taping*, the paper backing is torn in the middle with the effective area of the tape applied with medium stretch and the ends with no stretch.

**BUT:**

When applying a *Decompression Taping,* you apply the middle/effective area of the tape strip and then let go of it and apply one end after the other. Because the tape strip is stretched, the kinesiology tape will start to recoil the moment you let go of it and put down the ends.

When applying a *Stabilization Taping*, you want to reduce, if not avoid, the immediate recoil. You want to keep the original stretch of the tape, because this gives stability to the tissue underneath it!

So the tape is applied with a medium stretch, *but* you don't let go of it; instead, you instantly hold on to this part of the tape strip with a free hand/lower arm, keeping it in place with the stretch. With the other hand, you can then put down the ends one after the other, stretch-free as usual.

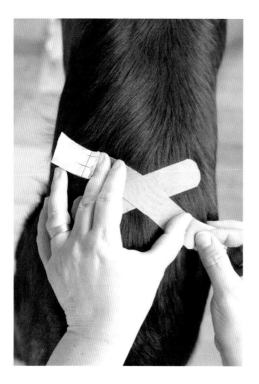

- Tear the paper backing off the first tape strip in the middle and remove it on both sides, until half an inch (1 cm) before the ends.

- Hold the tape strip with flat fingers on both ends, center it over the affected vertebrae at a 45-degree angle, and apply it with medium stretch.

- Immediately hold this section in place with one hand or have a helper hold on to it, to avoid the immediate recoil!

- While holding on to the effective area of the tape with one hand, you can now remove the paper backing from the ends and put these down, one after the other, stretch-free as usual.

- When the ends are fully applied, you can let go of the middle section.

*The active area of the tape strip is held in place immediately after the application and then the stretch-free ends are put on. This prevents the primary recoil and the remaining tension will give this body area more stability.*

- Rub over the tape vigorously but carefully, to activate the adhesive through frictional heat.

- Tear and remove the paper backing of the second tape strip as you did with the first one.

- Center this second tape strip over the affected vertebrae also, but angle it 45-degrees in the opposite direction, creating an X. Apply the tape and immediately hold on to the middle section to avoid the primary recoil.

- While holding down the effective part of the tape strip with one hand, remove the paper backing from each end and apply them without stretch and with a backup.

- Now you can let go of the middle section of the tape strip.

- Rub over the tape vigorously but carefully, to activate the adhesive through frictional heat.

*The complete application of a Stabilization Taping over a vertebra. The blue X is placed directly over the vertebra and the red strips are placed on the caudal and cranial joint space.*

- Tape strips three and four will be applied in the same manner, but they are placed parallel to the joint space, cranially and caudally of the affected vertebra.

- Rub over each tape strip individually to activate the adhesive.

The technique of applying the tape, holding onto the middle section immediately and then putting down the ends does take some practice. With this application, it is helpful to have assistance or get the dog owner involved by

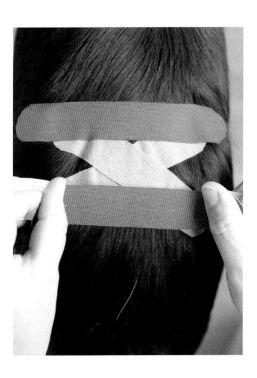

having him or her hold on to the tape. After the middle section (effective area) of the I-Tape has been applied, the helper can hold on to this part near both ends and keep it in place while you finish the application by putting down the ends stretch-free without having to hurry.

## Sacroiliac Joints

The technique is identical to the one mentioned above, only the positioning of the tape strips differs slightly, since the joints are running in a different direction.

For sacroiliac issues, the blue cross (the X) is centered directly over the sacrum, and the two red single I-Tapes are placed on the right and left sides of the sacrum since this is where the SI joints are located.

In this case, the X stabilizes the sacrum and the two single I-Tapes support the joint space of the sacroiliac joint.

*In the area of the sacrum and the sacroiliac joint, the X of the Stabilization Taping is positioned directly over the sacrum while the third and fourth tape strips are centered over the sacroiliac joints on the right and left side of the sacrum.*

## Stabilization Taping—Spine and Sacrum

**Direction of the tape:** from the inside out, keeping up the tension.
**Recoil:** while holding onto the tension, there is no recoil in this taping.
**Effect:** support for the stabilization of the vertebrae/sacrum while keeping up the tension. The cross (X) gives support to the vertebrae/sacrum, and the parallel strips stabilize the joint spaces.

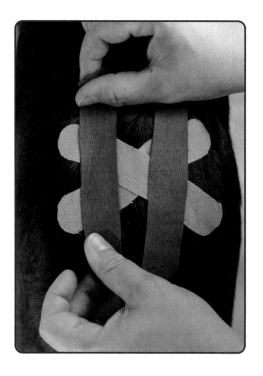

## Joints of the Extremities

Of course, you could also work on elbow or knee joints with the technique just mentioned, but this can be challenging due to the anatomy and range of motion in these areas. A lot of times, tape doesn't adhere well around these joints and their constant flexing compromises the taping application's longevity. A dog's elbow is difficult because it is mostly too close to the body/abdomen, and you just don't have enough area to tape to. On the other hand, the knee, with its wide range of motion and flexion, puts too much strain on this kind of application and this can cause an early detachment of the tape.

While this technique for the vertebrae works great on the carpal joint, we use a totally different type of *Stabilization Taping* for the knee and elbow. It is known as the front leg/hind leg *Sling Taping*.

For *Sling Taping*, you need a long I-Tape, which is applied using the *End-to-End* technique. The best way to apply this taping is while the dog is standing upright on all fours—in a relaxed stance—since you have to work your way around the leg with the tape.

**Example of a Hind-Leg *Sling Taping***

Start measuring a tape strip, beginning in the middle of the outside of the upper leg, then leading it forward and downward toward the knee, around the front of the knee (knee joint) to the inside of the leg, horizontally along the inner side of the leg and around the back of the knee. From there you go forward and upward back to the starting point where the tape strip can overlap slightly. When applying the tape, you work your way around the leg in the same direction.

- Tear the paper backing completely across about one inch (2 cm) from one end of the tape strip and remove it completely. Apply this primary end stretch-free at the point where you started your measurement.

- Remove the paper backing only piece by piece since the tape strip will be applied in segments.

- With a light stretch as it comes off the paper backing, the first section is applied from the primary end along the side of the leg forward and downward just until the outside edge of the knee.

- A second person should hold the tape in place at this point of the leg.

- Apply the next section with medium stretch around the knee joint from the lateral (outside) edge to the medial (inner) edge of the knee.

- Now your helper can let go of the first spot and hold the tape in place at this point of the leg.

- Tape horizontally along the inside of the leg with a light off-paper stretch just until the medial (inner) edge of the back of the knee.

- Your helper can now switch to this point of the leg and keep the tape in place.

- Apply the tape with medium stretch around the back of the knee from the medial side to the lateral side.

- Have your helper keep the tape in place at the lateral edge of the back of the knee. Then point your tape back to your starting place (primary end) and apply this last section with a light off-paper stretch until the last inch (2 to 3 cm).

- The secondary end should overlap with the primary end and has to be applied with no stretch.

- Rub over the tape carefully but vigorously to activate the adhesive through frictional heat.

Holding on to the tape and keeping it in place between segments helps to make a clear transition between the different sections of the tape and the different amounts of stretch.

This application requires some practice, a helper, and a dog that will

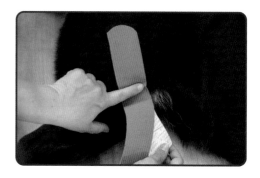

*The primary end of Sling Taping is applied in the middle of the upper leg on the lateral side of the dog's hind extremity. From there you work your way downward to the lateral side of the knee joint with a light stretch.*

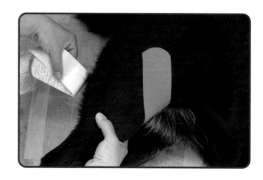

*After applying the tape with a medium stretch around the knee joint, continue horizontally on the inside of the leg with a light stretch to the medial side of the back of the knee.*

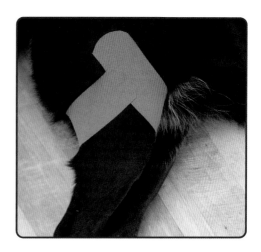

remain still for a few minutes! Since you are working with two different amounts of stretch in the tape strip (a medium stretch behind the knee and over the knee joint, and the rest with a light stretch) it is better to remove the paper backing piece by piece as needed for each segment at the time. Otherwise, this rather long piece of tape might suddenly attach somewhere else on the dog where it isn't supposed to!

On the front leg, a *Stabilization Taping* for the elbow joint can be applied in the same way. The *Sling Tape* gives more stability to the joint because related areas are applied with more tension, and at the same time, the whole extremity experiences an upward "lift" through the closed sling technique. It also addresses the dog's proprioception, improving body awareness and affects body stability.

*The back of the knee is taped with a medium stretch, and from there, the tape is brought upward again toward the primary end with a light stretch. The secondary end should overlap the primary end.*

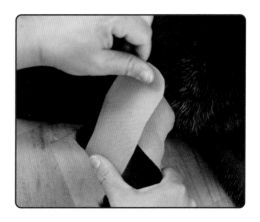

*The application of a Stabilization Taping for the elbow joint.*

# Tendon Taping

As previously explained, muscles are attached to bones through tendons at the origin and the insertion of the muscle. Muscles and muscle fibers are covered and sheathed by fascia. These connective-tissue fascia sheaths derive the parallel, organized tendon fibers, which look like whitish strands.

Tendons contain very few elastic fibers and, therefore, are very tensile- and tear-proof. Longer tendons such as the superficial, deep digital flexor and extensor tendons can have a certain but small amount of elasticity and spring force, because of their length. This helps to compensate for the excessive short-term strain of the tissue.

Constant overuse of an extremity, bad posture, and excessive strain can lead to chronic tendon strain or a tear, or even a partial or complete rupture of the tendon. You can use *Tendon Taping* as a preventive or rehabilitative tool when the dog is continuously overloading one extremity or has injured the tendon.

*Tendon Taping of the extensor tendon of the front leg. The muscle is taped along with the tendon. This gives you a combined and optimized effect along the muscle and tendon.*

## Application of a Tendon Taping

The actual part of the tendon that has "only" tendon fibers in the flexor and extensor tendons of dogs is located below the carpal joint of the front leg and below the tarsal joint of the hind leg. Above those areas you will find muscle and muscle fibers along with tendon fibers. The transition from muscle to tendon is very smooth in the dog's extremities. The muscle belly (see p. 66) also contains a lot of tendon fibers and segments, reaching into the actual tendon. Consequently, it is often difficult to differentiate muscle and tendon into two separate parts.

Also, depending on the breed of dog, the part below the carpal joint/tarsal joint can be really short, sometimes

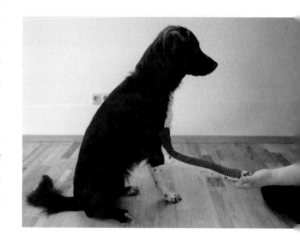

even too short to just tape the tendon by itself. So most of the time, it is better to start the *Tendon Taping* on the front leg below the shoulder or below the elbow. On the hind leg, it is best to start at the height of the knee, which is more than just a "pure" *Tendon Taping* since the application covers part of the muscle and muscle fibers as well. This is not a bad thing: if there is an injury to the tendon, the associated muscle is under strain as well in most cases, so it is advantageous for the muscle to be taped along with the tendon.

The general rule for a *Tendon Taping* is that the kinesiology tape is always applied from *proximal*, meaning closer to the body, toward *distal*, that is, toward the paw. This way, the recoil is always in the same direction as the contraction of the tendon and muscle. Most tendon injuries are a result

of overstretching the fibers. You never want to tape from *distal to proximal*, creating the recoil *toward* the paw, thereby causing the tendon to stretch even farther! It is this over-stretching of the tendon that you want to counteract. Therefore, always apply the tape from proximal to distal, to support the contraction of the muscle and tendon.

The *End-to-End* technique is used for a *Tendon Taping* and one single I-Tape is needed for this application. You have to measure from the elbow or the knee toward the paw as far as possible. The taping application should end just above the toes. The tape strip should be split lengthwise in the middle for smaller dogs or dogs with thin legs.

Pre-stretching the extremity is helpful in preparation for the actual application but not mandatory. So if you want to tape a flexor, gently bring the leg and paw straight forward as much as the dog will allow. For a taping on the extensor tendon, gently bring the leg backward and flex it, if the dog allows.

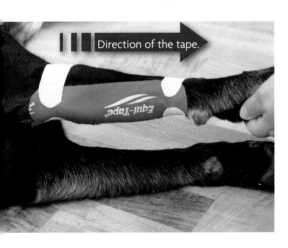

Direction of the tape.

*Since most tendon injuries are a result of an over-stretching in the distal direction, the tape is applied from proximal to distal, creating a recoil in the Tendon Tape, which is pointed proximally, thereby supporting the contraction of the tendon and the associated muscle.*

An assistant should hold the leg in this pre-stretched position until the application is completed.

- Tear the paper backing about 1 inch (2 cm) across from one end and remove it completely at this end.

- The primary end is applied with no stretch proximally at the height of the elbow, likewise the knee joint.

- Remove the paper backing until the last inch (2 cm) of the tape strip and aim it along the leg toward the paw.

- Hold the tape with flat fingers and give it a light to medium stretch. With this stretch, apply it evenly along the tendon.

- The last inch (2 cm) is applied as a stretch-free secondary end.

- Rub over the tape vigorously but carefully to activate the adhesive through frictional heat.

Due to the range of motion when flexing and extending the leg, while walking, running and so on, it is advisable to secure the application with horizontal stretch-free anchors.

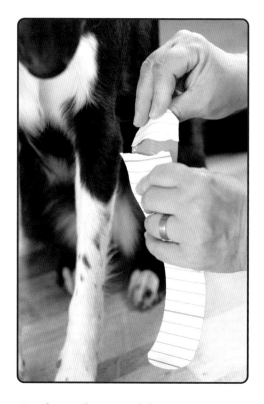

*For the application of the primary, cranial end, the paper backing is torn entirely across and removed about 1 inch (2 cm) from one end.*

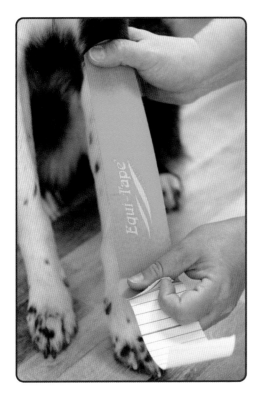 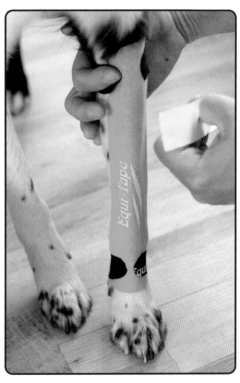

*After applying the stretch-free primary end, the tape strip is given a light to medium stretch, aimed toward the paw and then put down straight with the End-to-End technique. The secondary end is taped with no stretch.*

*Tendon Tapings should be secured with stretch-free cross-anchors, distal and proximal of the application.*

## Tendon Taping

**Direction of the tape:** in the distal direction, toward the paw.

**Recoil:** in the proximal direction, toward the body.

**Effect:** support of the tendon contraction and relief for the over-stretched fibers.

# Proprioception Taping

Proprioception has already been mentioned in the chapter about the effects of kinesiology tape on page 17. The word *proprioception* derives from two Latin words: *proprius*, meaning "own, one's own" and *recipere*, meaning "perceive, be aware of, take in." It describes the awareness of the body itself, its movement and position in its surroundings, and also the positioning of each body part in relation to the whole body. It is, therefore, often described as body or self-awareness. The proprioceptive stimulus is transmitted through specific signals from sensory receptor cells, called the "proprioceptors." These specialized receptors are constantly measuring the status of the body and the motion apparatus, as well as changes within the body system. Proprioceptors are found all over the body in the muscle cells, tendon fibers, ligaments, and fascia. Scientists estimate that about 60 percent of the specialized proprioceptors are located in the subcutaneous fascia. For this reason,

proprioception can be easily addressed and stimulated with kinesiology tape.

When the gait or posture of the animal is impaired, the use of *Proprioception Taping* is recommended. The impairment could be caused by damage to nerves and/or the nervous system, compression from a disc herniation, muscle atrophy, compensatory movement patterns, pain, injury—the list goes on.

## Application of a Proprioception Taping

For this application, a Fan-Tape is always used, and it needs an even

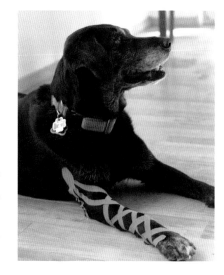

*The Proprioception Taping should encase and cover the entire extremity evenly, to stimulate it all over. The complete application often looks like the dog is wearing a fishnet stocking.*

number of fingers. The Fan-Tape is taped using the *End-to-End* technique.

An even number of fingers is necessary for the symmetry of the *Proprioception Taping*. Four fingers are usually the perfect amount; two are often not enough, and six, in most cases, are too many.

When taping the front leg, you have to measure from the shoulder joint, down the leg, all the way to the paw. On the hind leg, you start measuring from the hip joint all the way to the paw. Depending on the size of the dog, you have to add another 2 to 6 inches (5 to 15 cm) to the already measured length of your tape strip.

- Tear the paper backing apart at the transition from the primary end to each finger and fold the paper over.

- Remove the paper backing completely from the primary end and apply it with no stretch at the height of the shoulder or the hip.

- Take one of the outer fingers, remove a part of the paper backing, and hold this part of the tape so it is not dangling. The tape should not be stretched!

- In this un-stretched state, the tape is applied spiraling down around the leg toward the paw.

- Keep removing short sections of the paper backing, releasing the off-paper stretch, and working your way down the leg, in a spiral.

- Next, you use the other outside finger strip.

- With the same style and no stretch, this tape finger is also applied spiraling around the leg, but in the opposite direction.

- After the two outside tape strips have been applied, they should cross over each other at several points on the leg.

- Continue with the inner tape fingers, using the same method. Always release the 10 percent off-paper stretch.

- The right inner finger is applied parallel, just a little bit lower, to the outer right finger and also spiraling down around the leg.

- The left inner finger is applied parallel, just a little bit lower, to the outer left finger and spiraling around the leg.

*Fan-Tapes are always used for Proprioception Tapings. It has one closed primary end and an even number of fingers; four fingers are perfect. First, the paper backing is torn across at the transition between the primary end and each finger, and then it is completely removed at the end. The primary end is applied stretch-free.*

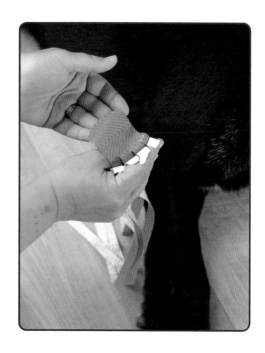

- All finger endings are, of course, applied without any stretch—as usual.

At the end, the whole extremity is spirally wrapped by the tape fingers, creating a grid-like pattern. After the Fan-Tape's complete application, it looks a bit like a fishnet stocking.

Since this application shouldn't have any stretch in the kinesiology tape, there should be no recoil as a result. It only creates a small impulse of shear motion for the sensory cells and the proprioceptor cells around the root of the hair when the dog is moving. But this tiny impulse is everywhere on the extremity since it is completely covered and encased by the grid

*The first outer finger is pointed cranio-distally and taped in a spiral around the extremity. The material is not stretched for this application!*

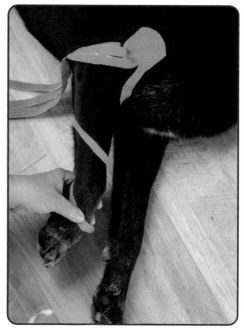

pattern. The proprioceptors are receiving the signal, "Watch out! There is something!" The body reacts to this impulse by activating the extremity, lifting it more, flexing it more, and thereby stimulating and strengthening the musculature.

It is always advisable to secure the thin finger endings with a horizontal, completely stretch-free cross-anchor.

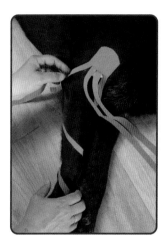 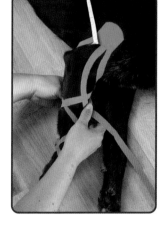 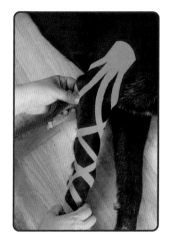

*The opposite outer-tape finger is pointed caudo-distally and also applied with almost no stretch spiraling around the leg in the opposite direction.*

*The inner cranial finger is applied spiraling parallel to the outer cranial finger, just a little bit lower. Again, there is hardly any stretch in the tape.*

*At last, the inner caudal finger is applied: spiraling around the leg, parallel to the outer caudal finger, and stretch-free.*

## Proprioception Taping

**Direction of the Tape:** spiraling distally toward the paw, but without stretch.

**Recoil:** since the whole application is applied stretch-free, there is no recoil.

**Effect:** supports body awareness by stimulating the proprioceptors through shear motion between the tape and hair/root when the dog is moving.

# Cross Tapes

Now I want to introduce a kinesiology tape specialty: *Cross Tapes*. These tapes are also called *Cross Patches* or *Grid Tape*. Their fabric is made of a cotton-silk mixture. But in contrast to the kinesiology tape rolls, they don't have any elastic fibers so they are not flexible and can't be stretched. *Cross Tapes* are made with a similar acrylic adhesive, are non-medicated, and are available in different sizes. Their unique feature is that they are statically charged; in fact, they are charged as a result of the cotton-silk fabric being removed from the paper backing.

Like the *Cross Tapes*, your skin, as well as a dog's hair, are statically charged. Injury, sickness, or any disorder of the tissue or energy flow can change the acid-base environment;

therefore, the static charge on the surface of that area can change as well. Through the specific pattern of the *Cross Tapes*, the decompressing effect on the tissue is very tiny. Still, it regulates and normalizes the static charge of the affected area through the static charge of the *Cross Tape*. This stimulates and regulates energy flow and also supports pain relief.

*Cross Tapes* can be used in conjunction with kinesiology tape or used separately. They are usually used for particular problems in small areas, such as trigger points, stress points, or focal points of pain. Their most common use is the treatment of acupuncture points to support acupuncture, acupressure, or laser-acupuncture treatments.

*Cross Tapes, also called Grid Tapes or Cross Patches, are available in different sizes. For treating acupuncture points, the small ones are most suitable.*

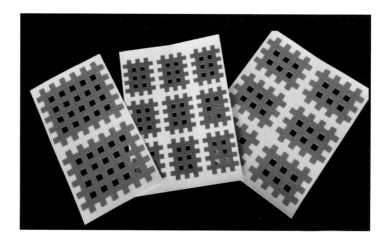

## The Application of Cross Tapes

- Carefully get hold of the *Cross Tape* on one corner with your fingertips or tweezers and remove it from the paper backing.

- Hold on to the *Cross Tape* at just this one corner. This way, your own static charge will not "interfere" with the static charge of the *Cross Tape*.

- With just a tiny air gap between hair and tape, slide the *Cross Tape* carefully over the hair in the affected area.

- Through the change in the static charge of the skin/hair, the *Cross Tape* will find the affected spot by itself.

- The *Cross Tape* pulls toward the affected point in the hair and adheres on its own.

- **Do not rub over the *Cross Tape*!** You risk rubbing the small *Cross Tape* off accidentally and potentially changing the static charge by rubbing it, which is not desirable in this application.

*Cross Tapes*, like kinesiology tape, can stay on the hair as long as they are needed. They will fall off when their "job" is done. Some can fall off after 24 hours, while others stay on longer. I have had *Cross Tapes* that didn't come off for 10 days. If you have a dog with hair that requires grooming, you should carefully brush around the *Cross Tapes*.

*To avoid interfering with the static charge of the Cross Tapes, they should be held at only one corner. Tweezers can be a helpful tool here. The Cross Tapes are held close over the hair. Due to the static charge, they will pull toward the affected area and onto the hair by themselves and attach there.*

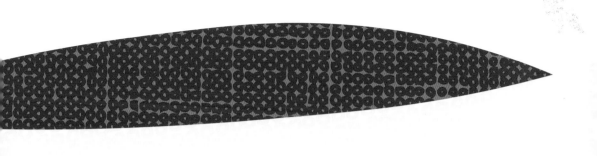

# Chapter 6:
# Case Studies from My
# Physiotherapy Practice

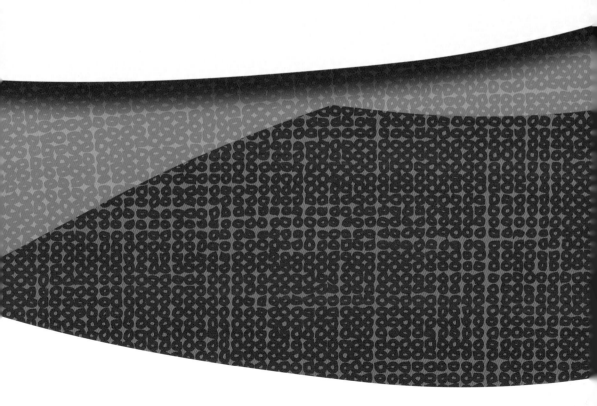

In this chapter, I would like to share some case studies from my daily practice. These cases will demonstrate the many taping patterns as well as address some common conditions and how they can be combined with physiotherapy work.

Many of these cases were conducted with my colleague Jennifer Born and made available with the friendly support of generous dog owners. I thank all involved for this great collaboration and the support I had in putting these together.

# Strain of the Flexor Tendon and Distortion of the Carpal Joint

**Case History:** Seven-Year-Old Labrador, Female

Unfortunately, this dog had a nasty slip during her work as a rescue dog and sprained her left front leg. In the beginning, she was obviously lame and only walked on the tip of her toes.

**Physical Therapy:** Massage and passive movement of the left overstretched front leg, along with manual therapy and osteopathic techniques to release the distortion and blockage in the carpal joint. This treatment was repeated several times during a period of two

months. After that, the dog showed no more signs of lameness.

**Taping Application:** A *Decompression Taping* was applied on the cranial side of the carpal joint. This

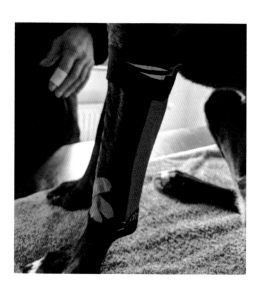

*A combined Muscle-Tendon Taping along the flexor tendon using cross-anchors at the proximal and distal end. In addition, a Decompression Taping was applied on the cranial side of the carpal joint.*

was combined with a *Tendon Taping* along the flexor tendon, which was secured proximally and distally with cross-anchors. The dog tolerated the application well and the tape was removed by the owner after two days.

# Unclear Lameness with Tension in the M. latissimus dorsi

**Case History:** Ten-Year-Old Jack Russell Terrier, Male

The dog was showing a rather stiff gait on the right front leg. During palpation, the joints of this leg proved to be rather stiff with minimal flexion—arthrosis was suspected. The *M. latissimus dorsi* was very tight.

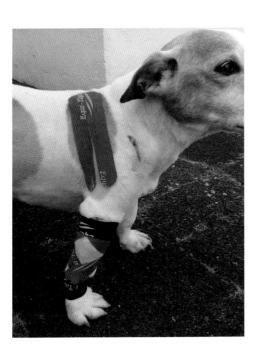

**Physical Therapy:** Whole body massage with focus on the right *M. latissimus dorsi*. Careful passive movement and stretching of the right front leg. Magnetic blanket treatment. The owner was advised to have the dog rest with a heating pad in his dog bed.

**Taping Application:** After releasing tension out of the muscle, a *Muscle Taping* to support and activate the *M. latissimus dorsi* was applied. In addition, a *Proprioception Taping* was applied on the right front leg to raise and improve body awareness in the leg.

The dog tolerated the tape very well, but unfortunately, it became loose after one day. While the dog was taped, he showed an improvement in his gait and less stiff in the leg. The application

*Combination of a Muscle Taping for the M. longissimus dorsi with a Proprioception Taping on the right front leg.*

was repeated once. Before applying the tape, the area was thoroughly wiped down with baby powder to reduce the skin's oiliness. The second application stayed on for several days.

# Back Pain and Uneven Gait

**Case History:** Six-Year-Old Mixed Breed, Female

The dog had shown an uneven gait for quite some time; the hind legs were placed laterally to the right compared to the front legs. When the dog started having trouble getting up and began to walk out of rhythm, the knee seemed to be falling out to the side. After visiting the veterinarian and getting an X-ray, it showed that the acetabulum of the hip joint was very flat and short and that the femoral head did not sit in the socket. The dog was also very pain-reactive in her back, and the X-ray showed that the last lumbar vertebra was tilted ventrally and slightly to the right.

**Physical Therapy:** Manual therapy of the lumbar spine to correct the positioning of the last lumbar vertebra, and relaxing massage for the hypertonic lumbar muscles followed by a magnetic blanket session. Mobilization of the

pelvis as well as activating massage of the thigh adductor muscles and relaxing massage of the thigh abductor muscles.

**Taping Application:** A hind-leg *Sling Taping* was applied to give the hind leg, especially the knee, more stability. After physiotherapy and application of the tape, the gait immediately showed improvement and the knee didn't

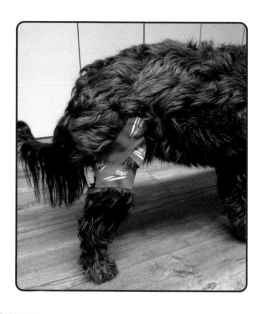

*Hind-leg Sling Taping to stabilize the hind extremity.*

rotate so much to the outside any-more. The dog tolerated the tape, and it remained for a week. After that time, it was carefully removed by the owner.

# Complete Biceps Tendon Tear of the Left Front Leg

**Case History:** Four-Year-Old Mixed Breed, Female

Three months prior to starting the physiotherapy, while out for a walk and playing with other dogs, this dog suddenly seemed to be in pain and was lame on the left front leg. An immediate visit to the veterinarian did not give any clear diagnosis. After several visits to different vets and numerous examinations, a complete tear of the biceps tendon was diagnosed. By then it was too late for surgery, according to the veterinarian's report. Instead, she was given a sling to wear during the day to give the shoulder and front leg more protection and stability.

**Physical Therapy:** To reduce the pain in the injured leg, the dog compensated by shifting her weight more and more onto the right front leg, and as a result, this extremity was overworked and became tight. There was also some tension in the right hind leg, again from shifting her weight diagonally away from the injured leg. A gentle, relaxing massage of all overworked body parts as well as stretching exercises for the right front and hind leg. An activating massage on the left front leg and passive movement of all joints in the front leg.

*Muscle-Tendon Taping for the biceps tendon with multiple cross-anchors.*

Right after the tape was applied, the dog received a therapeutic session in the water treadmill to help strengthen the left front leg.

**Taping Application:** After the physiotherapy and before going to water treadmill therapy, a combined *Muscle-Tendon Taping* was applied on the biceps muscle and tendon. The application was secured with multiple cross-anchors. After the water treadmill session, the shoulder support sling was put on over the tape. The dog tolerated the tape well on the first two days, but on the third day, she started chewing on it. The owner removed the application. The physiotherapy, water treadmill, and taping were repeated several times.

# Dragging Gait of the Left Hind Leg After a Disc Herniation Operation

**Case History:** One-Year-Old Australian Shepherd, Male

The dog had a disc herniation, which was successfully taken care of with surgery. Due to the compression of the nerve, prior to the operation, the dog developed a dragging, sluggish gait in the left hind leg. Even after the successful operation the dog continued to drag his leg.

**Physical Therapy:** Passive movement of the extremity and tapping massage to stimulate the nerve cells in the affected leg. The owner was advised to

*Proprioception Taping (with cranial and caudal cross-anchors) because of a dragging, sluggish gait in the left hind leg.*

actively look for tiny obstacles when taking the dog for a walk in the woods and have him walk over small branches

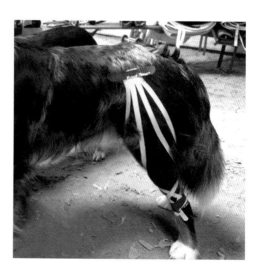

to activate the muscles in the hind leg. Treatment with the magnetic blanket and/or the water treadmill was recommended.

**Taping Application:** A *Proprioception Taping* was applied to the affected left hind leg. The primary end and the finger endings were secured with anchors. The gait started improving within a few minutes. As long as the dog was busy walking and getting attention from his owner, he tolerated the tape and it adhered well to his long hair. As soon as the dog was no longer distracted and left unattended, he started chewing on the tape and within an hour he had removed it entirely.

# Tension in the Sacrum Area and Reduced Mobility in the Sacroiliac Joints

**Case History:** Seven-Year-Old Hound/European Sled Dog, Male

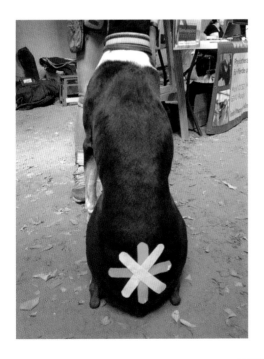

This dog was very active and participated in dogsledding, skijoring, bikejoring, and canicross competition. After a very intense training session the dog was very stiff in the hind legs and not eager to move anymore. The gluteal muscles were very tight and sore, and the sacroliac joints were compromised in their mobility and didn't swing through as they normally should.

**Physical Therapy:** Massage of the lumbar and gluteal area, as well as stretching. Mobilization of the pelvis with manual therapy and osteopathic

*Decompression Taping over the sacrum area.*

techniques. Daily treatment with a heating blanket or warm water bottle around the affected area for a few days was recommended to the owner.

**Taping Application:** *Decompression Taping* directly over the area of the sacrum and the sacroiliac joints to relieve some of the tension and pressure there. The taping application stayed on for three days and was then removed by the owner.

# Scar Taping After Surgical Removal of a Mast Cell Tumor

**Case History:** Six-Year-Old Australian Shepherd, Female

While casually petting her dog, the owner found a bulge under the skin in the area of the cranial part of the thoracic spine. The dog was taken to the vet to be examined. The tumor was surgically removed and the biopsy showed that it was a mast cell tumor.

**Physical Therapy:** Four days after the sutures had all been removed by the vet and the scabs had fallen off by themselves, the scar tissue was soft and mobile. An actual scar treatment and a massage weren't needed.

**Taping Application:** *Scar Taping* crosswise on the surgical scar. The application remained on the dog for three days. The owner removed it after the dog had excessively rolled in sand and the application looked really worn out.

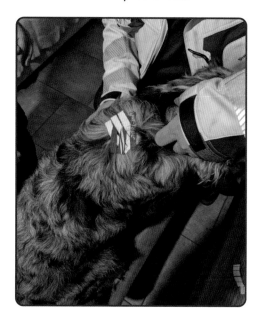

*Post-surgery Scar Taping after the removal of a mast cell tumor.*

# Muscle Atrophy of the Back Muscles and Misalignment of the Sacroiliac Joint

**Case History:** Ten-Year-Old Pug, Male

The little pug had multiple pre-existing illnesses. Ten days previous to the treatment he had a total physical break down, and it took him 10 minutes until he could get up again. He also hadn't been sleeping well since he couldn't find a comfortable position. His gait and posture analysis showed a lateral flexion of the spine to the right at the transition between the thoracic and lumbar spine. It also showed that

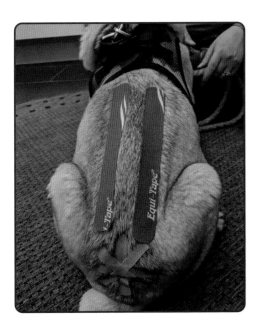

the right hind leg had rotated outward. During the manual palpation, the back muscle appeared very atrophic and misalignment could be found at the 10th thoracic vertebra, as well as in the right sacroiliac joint.

**Physical Therapy:** Activating massage of the back muscles as well as the gluteal muscles with a focus on the right gluteal and hind leg muscles. Releasing the misalignments of the spine and the pelvis through manual therapy and osteopathic techniques, along with mobilization of these areas afterward. The dog was also scheduled at a dog physiotherapy office the next week for a water treadmill session.

**Taping Application:** *Bilateral Muscle Taping* to activate the back muscles combined with a *Decompression Taping* over the sacrum and the sacroiliac joints.

*A combination of a back Muscle Taping with a Decompression Taping over the area of the sacroiliac joints.*

The tape remained on the dog for four days and was then removed by the owner, prior to going into his water treadmill session. During these four days, the dog slept a lot better because he was able to lie down more comfortably again.

# Tear of the Caudal Cruciate Ligament and Surgical Intervention

**Case History:** Two-Year-Old Mixed Breed, Male

This dog came from abroad and was kept in a small crate most of the time. Due to the lack of movement and exercise, the dog's muscles were all underdeveloped. He also had a deformity of the left tibia. The combination of these problems caused a rupture of the caudal cruciate ligament. Surgery repaired the rupture and an osteotomy of the tibia plateau was done to even out the deformity of the bone.

**Physical Therapy:** The dog received his first physiotherapy session shortly after the surgery. The area around the left knee was carefully massaged and moved passively by the therapist. The back muscles were still tight and received a relaxing massage. With ongoing physiotherapy and improvement in the range of motion, more exercises were added, such as "bicycle-riding motion" of the leg and walking over small obstacles. To strengthen the musculature,

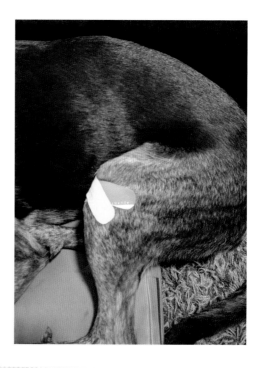

*Stabilization Taping over the gap of the knee joint.*

the dog also had sessions in the water treadmill in between.

The dog responded really well to the physiotherapy and showed an improvement in his gait and posture and started building up muscles quickly.

# Patellar Luxation

**Case History:** Five-Year-Old Mixed Breed, Female

This dog showed a constant patellar luxation toward the medial side. The dislocated kneecap would not return to its normal position. The dog was not bearing any weight on the affected leg. With surgery, the kneecap was put back into its normal position, and the overstretched ligaments were shortened.

**Taping Application:** *Stabilization Taping* over the space in the knee joint. The dog, who was rather cautious and scared easily, felt a little uncomfortable about the tape for the first few minutes, but then got used to it and tolerated it very well.

**Physical Therapy:** Physiotherapy began three weeks after the operation. In the beginning, the focus was on relaxing the overworked tissue in her back and the compensating legs. Exercises to strengthen the muscles in the healing leg and careful passive movement to restore the range of motion in the joint. Later, stabilization exercises

*Muscle Taping along the M. biceps femoris muscle to strengthen the lateral muscles on the upper leg and a Stabilization Taping lateral of the knee joint to help keep the patella in place.*

were added as well as aquatic therapy and working with obstacles.

**Taping Application:** A *Stabilization Taping* (yellow) was applied laterally to the knee joint, to help prevent the kneecap from falling out of the normal position to the medial side again. This was combined with a *Muscle Taping* (purple) along the *biceps femoris* muscle with a lateral recoil.

The fingers of the *Muscle Taping* were applied above and below the patella all the way around the knee to the inside of the leg. Over four weeks, this application was applied weekly and it always stayed on for two to three days. With the progressing physiotherapy and building of muscles, the extremity got more and more stable, and the dog began to stand normally. No further applications were needed.

# Hip Joint Arthrosis

**Case History:** Nine-Year-Old Golden Retriever, Female

The dog was showing more and more stiffness in her movement of the right hind leg. The owner was referring to it as her "peg leg." In particular, walking on very smooth surfaces, like hardwood or tiled floors, was becoming more and more difficult for her. An X-ray showed a clear image of arthrosis in her hip joint.

**Physical Therapy:** Along with anti-inflammatory and analgesic medication, the dog was treated with a thorough massage of the hind leg and a warm

water bottle. The therapist passively activated the hip joint. Still the dog was having trouble with the hip joint.

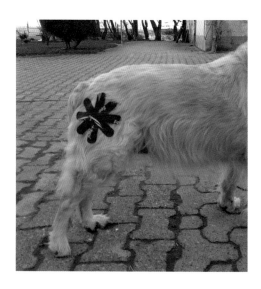

*Decompression Taping for a chronic arthrosis of the hip joint.*

To make it easier on the hip, slower and more controlled walks were suggested, despite her love of romping around in fields.

**Taping Application:** *Decompression Taping* over the hip joint. Through the decompressing effect, the pressure in the hip joint was reduced. After a few yards, the dog's movement—and especially the hind leg—improved and looked less stiff. The tape remained on the dog for a week and was repeated occasionally.

# Back Pain

**Case History:** Six-Year-Old Mixed Breed, Male

The dog was very uncomfortable and sore in his back and showed signs of

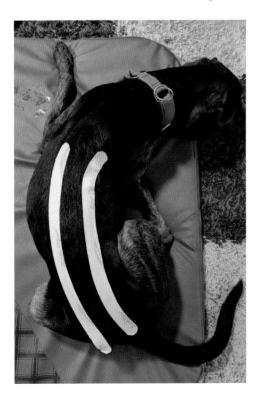

pain, a lot of tension in the area, and an overall stiff gait. X-rays showed that the dog had arthrosis in his lumbar spine, which led to a narrowing of the spinal cord.

**Physical Therapy:** Lots and lots of massage and stretching exercises. He did not like the treatment with the heating pad and always moved away. Instead, the magnetic blanket was used.

**Taping Application:** *Muscle Taping* on both sides along the spine, taped from cranial to caudal to relax the long back muscle. The application stayed on for several days and was repeated regularly with the physiotherapy.

*Bilateral Muscle Taping of the back for tight and painful muscles.*

# Unbalanced Posture with Lateral Body Flexion to the Right

**Case History:** Two-Year-Old Mixed Breed, Female

This dog was raised abroad under poor conditions, most likely always confined in a crate. The dog always walked in small circles, bending to the right. When asked to walk straight, the hind legs were clearly offset to the right as compared to the front legs. The body was twisted and bent to the right.

**Physical Therapy:** An X-ray showed deformity and multiple malformations along the spine. Some vertebrae showed signs of fusing and could not visibly be separated.

Along with massage, fascia techniques, and some stretching (when possible), the dog was treated with

*Fascia Tapings (red) with primary ends cranial and caudal, pointing the recoil in these directions, to help elongate the shortened fibers.*

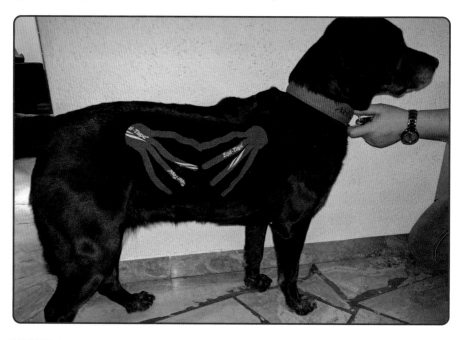

the magnetic blanket daily for several weeks. The body structures on the right side were shortened and restricted, and they were overstretched on the left side. So the goal was to get the dog a little bit straighter.

**Taping Application:** Application of *Fascia Tapings* on both sides of the body. On the right/shortened side, the tape (red) was applied from cranial and caudal to the center of the body,

*Additional Fascia Taping (blue) on the overstretched side with the primary ends in the middle, pointing the recoil to the center of the body to help contraction and shortening of the elongated side.*

thereby creating a recoil toward the head and the tail and helping to elongate the shortened side.

On the left/overstretched side, the tape (blue) was applied from the center of the body toward the head and the tail. This created a recoil to the center of the body to help shorten the overstretched fibers.

The *Fascia Tapings* on the right and left side were applied at the same time and these tapings were alternated with a *Back Muscle Taping*. Over a month, the applications were repeated multiple times during the physiotherapy sessions and the dog tolerated them without any problem.

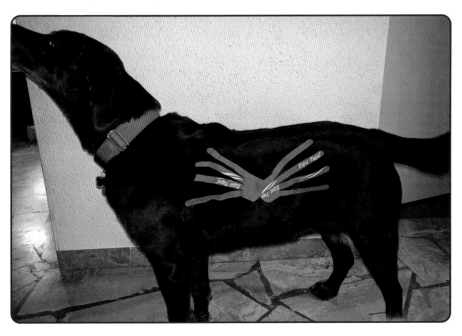

# Spondylosis and Arthrosis in the Lumbar Spine (Causing Trouble with Defecation)

**Case History:** Eight-Year-Old Cocker Spaniel, Male

When squatting down to defecate, the dog had trouble with his posture because he couldn't flex his back in this position. Since he was showing severe back pain and had trouble flexing his back, the veterinarian took an X-ray. It showed severe signs of spondylosis in the thoracic and lumbar spine as well as distinct arthrosis and osteophytes along the transverse processes of the lumbar vertebrae.

**Physical Therapy:** Going up and down stairs as well as jumping up or down were to be avoided. Intermittent medicinal leech therapy along the spine on both sides showed an improvement in gait and posture. In between the leech therapy sessions, the dog's back was massaged regularly, and he received magnetic blanket sessions.

**Taping Application:** *Stabilization Taping* along the thoracic and lumbar spine with additional cross-anchors at the ends. The dog tolerated the tape well, and it remained for three days before being removed by the owner. Whenever the gait and posture problems returned, the application was repeated.

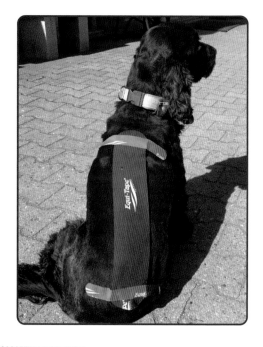

*Variation of a Stabilization Taping along the thoracic and lumbar spine because multiple segments and vertebrae were affected.*

# Cauda Equina Syndrome

**Case History:** Ten-Year-Old Mixed Breed, Female

The dog appeared more and more lethargic and unwilling to walk. The owner thought it was due to her advanced age. When she started dragging her toes on both hind legs, an X-ray was taken, followed by an MRI. They showed signs of degeneration on the last lumbar vertebra and the first sacral vertebra, with a stenosis of the spinal cord in that area and compression of the *cauda equina* fibers and nerves.

**Physical Therapy:** To avoid further irritation of the nerves and *cauda equina* fibers, a major cutback in the dog's daily activity and movement was advised. Analgesic and anti-inflammatory medications were prescribed. Physical therapy started with a gentle massage around the painful back. Then laser therapy was added, and after several weeks, a few minutes on the water treadmill.

**Taping Application:** *Decompression Taping* over the stenosis of the lumbosacral junction. The dog tolerated the tape well and it remained on for three days. The application was shown and explained to the owner, who independently repeated it at home by herself. The tape was applied weekly and stayed on for three to four days.

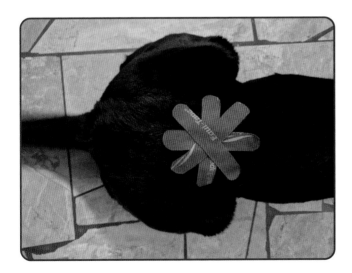

*Decompression Taping over the area of the lumbosacral joint to decompress the stenosis and reduce the tension on nerves and fibers.*

# Congenital Deformity of the Front Leg and Operation for Posture Correction

**Case History:** Eleven-Month-Old Bernese Mountain Dog / Poodle Mix, Male

The dog always showed a rather clumsy gait, but the owners put that down to his young age. But, when clipping his long curly hair in the summer, the deformity of the front leg, which had been completely hidden under the really long, thick, fluffy, and curly hair, became visible. The dog was taken to the veterinarian and X-rays were taken. A corrective osteotomy was done.

**Physical Therapy:** Immediately after the surgery, physical therapy started with massage and passive movement and stretching. It was repeated bi-weekly. Due to the massiveness of the deformity, a second surgery was done three month later with a double radius osteotomy. The bone was fixed in the new position with a plate and several screws (see X-ray on facing page). Unfortunately, the plate did not stay in place and broke off three days after the operation. Another surgery was done to reattach the plate onto the bone again.

After the third surgery, the affected paw was numb and didn't show any reflexes. No weight was put on this leg when walking so it was mostly just "dangling" from the elbow. A special arrhythmical massage was done repeatedly to stimulate the nerves and muscles in the extremity, with minimal improvement.

**Taping Application:** *Muscle Tendon* tapings were applied 14 days after the third operation to support the posture correction of the extremity. The front leg still showed a slight outward rotation, causing the medial side still to be overstretched and the lateral side shortened. The medial side was taped from proximal to distal with medium stretch (yellow tape) to create a recoil going proximally and to support the overstretched side's contraction. The lateral side was taped from distal to proximal with medium stretch (green tape), creating a recoil distally to help stretch the shortened side. When leaving the physiotherapist's office, the dog tried to put weight onto that leg and the numb paw for the first time! Unfortunately, the application only lasted for three hours, because the dog started chewing on it when he got bored. But within those first three hours, the gait had noticeably improved.

The application was repeated during the weekly physiotherapy sessions and, over time, the dog tolerated it better and it lasted longer. The owner put a long-sleeved shirt on the dog after the tape was applied so that the dog could not reach it and chew on it.

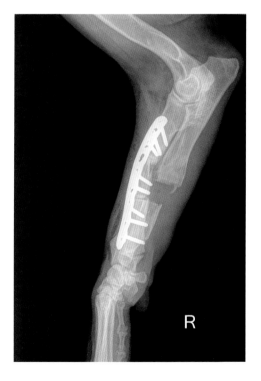

*An X-ray after corrective osteotomy of the front leg with a plate and multiple screws.*

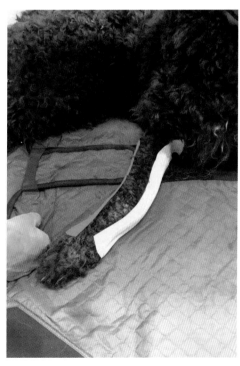

*Muscle-Tendon Taping to help support posture correction. The yellow tape has a recoil pointed cranially and the green tape has recoil pointed distally.*

# Lameness of the Right Hind Leg (Suspected Herniated Disc and Cruciate Ligament Tear)

**Case History:** Fourteen-Year-Old Shih Tzu, Female

After taking a walk, the dog was suddenly lame on the right hind leg and could hardly put any weight on it. The gait was compromised and the leg was "thrown" forward. A controlled forward movement of the leg was not possible anymore. Since the dog could not put her weight onto that leg it was very difficult for her to urinate or defecate. A vet visit lead to the suspected diagnosis of a herniated disc in the lumbar area, and a cruciate ligament tear in the right hind leg. Due to

the age of the dog and other multiple pre-existing illnesses, an operation was not an option.

**Physical Therapy:** Start of physiotherapy about a week after the diagnosis from the vet. The muscles on the right hind leg were already clearly atrophic. The leg was still not weight-bearing. An activating massage to stimulate the musculature of that leg and passive movement of hip and knee joints.

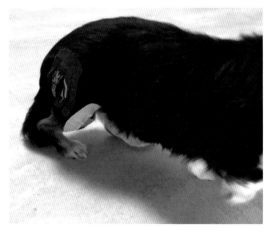

*Muscle Taping using a Fan-Tape to activate the musculature of the hind leg. This was combined with a Stabilization Taping for the knee and patella.*

Gentle stroking massage along the lower part of the leg to stimulate proprioception along with stabilization exercises. The magnetic blanket was rented out to the dog owner, allowing the dog daily magnetic blanket sessions. At the second appointment, a week later, the situation was unchanged.

**Taping Application:** During the second appointment, the dog was also taped along with the actual physiotherapy work. A *Muscle Taping* for the hind leg musculature was applied (red tape), as was a *Stabilization Taping* directly over the knee gap (green tape) and laterally and medially around the patella (yellow tape). After about five minutes, the dog started showing signs of improvement in her gait, putting a little weight on that leg. She could get a better grip on the smooth floor and the paw didn't always slip away. The kinesiology tape remained on the dog for four days and the owner called on the first evening to report that the dog could stand a lot better and was more stable when "going to the bathroom."

During the next physiotherapy appointment, a *Stabilization Tape* was applied to the lumbosacral area and a *Proprioception Taping* along the right hind extremity. This brought a noticeable improvement in the gait and posture and remained on the dog for four days. A week later, you could clearly see an improvement in the musculature of the right hind leg and that it was getting stronger. This second set of applications was repeated multiple times.

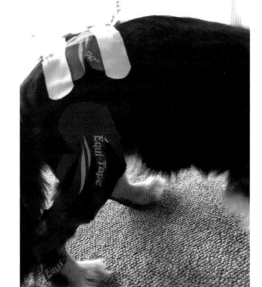

*A combination of a Proprioception Taping on the hind leg and a Stabilization Taping over the pelvis.*

# About the Author

Several years ago, an issue with my own horse led me to physical therapy for horses, since the veterinarian couldn't help, but the physical therapist could.

During my time of study to become an animal Physical Therapist (PT), I watched the Olympic summer games, and that is when I first saw athletes (mainly beach volleyball players and track competitors) wearing these colorful stripes on their bodies. Of course, I wanted to know what this was about, and I started gathering information about taping. At that time, it wasn't so easy since taping wasn't popular yet. But I could find information on the subject, and I thought that this could work on animals as well. After some thorough research, I found a course for equine kinesiology taping. I took this course along with my regular PT classes. That was the beginning of it all, and as soon as I started practicing it with my own horse and he was seen walking around the arena in his colorful stripes, people naturally started asking about it.

A few years ago we had to move from Germany to the United States because of my husband's work, and that is when I met the Equi-Tape® company.

Their CEO at that time came to a taping demonstration of mine, and I took a course with Dr. Beverly Gordon, the developer and founder of Equi-Tape®, which was the first tape to be especially designed just for the use on horses.

Over time, I met a lot of fellow animal practitioners in Germany and in the United States who had taping experience. I also took other courses with different instructors. Ideas and taping applications were exchanged. There was a lot of trial and error in my own experiences before I finally found my way of taping. And now my taping applications have good longevity and results that I can recommend. I have held countless demonstrations for therapist and animal owners. When we moved back to Germany a few years ago, I became the sole distributor for Equi-Tape® in my home country.

Again and again, clients asked me to write a book about this subject, since I could always explain it in a clear way that was easy to understand.

Since the majority of my patients are horses and horse taping is more common than dog taping, I put my focus on them and my first book *Kinesiologisches Pferdetaping* was published in German by Müller Rüschlikon Verlag in 2016. The English translation *Kinesiology Taping for Horses* by Trafalgar Square Books followed in 2018.

But people kept approaching me about a book specifically written for taping dogs. So *Kinesiologisches Taping für Hunde* was published by Kynos Verlag in 2019, followed by the English version in 2020, again by Trafalgar Square Books.

# Contact

If you have any further questions about *Kinesiology Taping* for dogs or horses, you can go to my website
www.horse-wellness.com

or visit my Facebook and Instagram pages for more information.
www.facebook.com/horsewellnessllc/
www.instagram.com/
katjashorsewellness/

Or just send me an email at
katja@horse-wellness.com

For Equi-Tape® orders go to:
www.equi-tape.com
www.equi-tape.de (Germany and Europe)

Other kinesiology tapes I have used that are also featured in this book include:
Rock Tape® www.rocktape.com
Spidertech™ www.spidertech.com

# Recommended Resources

*Dog Anatomy Workbook: A Guide to the Canine Body*
Andrew Gardiner and Maggie Raynor
ISBN: 9781570766961 (Trafalgar Square Books)

*Gymnastricks*
Carmen Mayer
ISBN: 9781910488423 (Corpus Publishing Limited)

*The Healthy Way to Stretch Your Dog: A Physical Therapy Approach*
Sasha Foster and Ashley Foster
ISBN: 9781929242542 (Dogwise Publishing)

*Canine Massage—A Complete Reference Manual*
Jean-Pierre Hourdebaigt
ISBN: 9781929242085 (Dogwise Publishing)

*Canine Rehabilitation and Physical Therapy*
David Levine and Darryl L. Millis
ISBN: 9781437703092 (Saunders)

# Acknowledgments

A lot is needed to write a book—especially support. I could never have done this all by myself. The biggest supporter and helper, as always, is my husband. He fully supports all my activities and helps me whenever he can. He is my first reader, and he takes the photos, creates diagrams, and, and, and…. He comes up with new ideas and input when I get stuck and don't know how to continue. Thank you so much, Robert. I wouldn't know how to do this without you.

I would like to thank my two dear colleagues, Kathelijne Hornix and Jennifer Born (www.tierphysio-jenni-fer-born.de) for their support in this book's creation. They have provided me with case studies from their daily physiotherapy practice. I love our dinner meetings with lots of talk about animal physiotherapy. Jenny's support and patience during various photo shoots were worth a fortune. Thank you, Jenny, for all your help with the pictures for this book.

Of course, a big, big thank you goes to our two four-legged supermodels, Maja and Abby. They did a fabulous job sitting or lying around, modeling for this book more or less patiently. I have to tell you: a great deal can be achieved with the help of dog treats! Maja can now work as a professional model. At our first photo shoot, she was obviously confused and a little bit stressed about what we wanted her to do and why she should sit, stand, or lie in a specific position. At our final shoot, I just had to get the tape and the treats out, and she immediately sat down and put herself in a good taping position.

I would also like to thank all the other dogs who have been taped so willingly and became models for this book. And thank you to all their owners for letting me work on their dogs and giving me permission to make them part of this book.

Like my first book in English (*Kinesiology Taping for Horses*) my dear friend Jenny Stieglitz from www.savvycanine-equinetraining.com and her mother Francine Stieglitz were involved, reading through my German-English translation, making sure everything could be understood. Thanks for all your work. You are the best.

I would like to thank Kynos Verlag and Gisela Rau for the German version and Trafalgar Square Books and Martha Cook for the English version of this book and for supporting the idea and making my project come true.

Thanks to everyone who was involved in the book's making.

# Index

Page numbers in *italics* indicate illustrations.

Frictional heat, in activation of adhesive, 11, 49–50, *49*
Fungal infections, 30
Fur. *See* Hair/fur

Gait abnormalities
    case studies, 18, 119–123, 125–27, 129, 132, 134–37
    taping techniques for, 15, 73, 110
Goethe, Johann Wolfgang von, 19
Green, color effects, 22
Grid application, of Lymphatic Tapings, 79, *79*
Grid Tape, 114–15, *114–15*

Hair/fur
    length of, 32–33, 37–38
    preparation of, 36
    sensation and, 8
    tape adhesion and, 9–10, 12–13, 38
Healing, of wounds, 30. *See also* Scar tissue
Hematoma Tapings, 44, 96–98, *97–98*
Hips
    case studies, 120–21
    dysplasia in, taping benefits, 15
Hygiene considerations, 30, 36
Hypersensitivities, 31–32
Hypertonic muscles, 61
Hypertrophic muscles, 62
Hypotonic muscles, 61

Indications, for taping, 26–29
Infections, 31
Inflammation, 15
Insertion site, of muscles, 61, 66
Inside-Out Taping technique
    described, 45, *45*
    recoil in, 63
    uses of, 82, 92
Irritation risk, 31–32, 52
I-Tape cuts
    described, 43, *43*
    uses of, 80, 85, 92, 99, 103, 107

Joints
    anchoring tapings near, 53
    instability in, 28
    misalignment/blocking in, 92
    support of, 16–17, *16*, 103–5

Kase, Kenzo, 2–3, 5
Kinesiology, generally, 5–6
Kinesiology Tape
    adhesiveness of, 9–10, *10*, 12–13
    application and handling of, 46–55
    benefits, 15–18
    characteristics of, 8–13
    color of, 11, 19–23, *19*
    history of, 2–5
    measurement of, 68, *69*
    misapplication of, 50
    preparation of, 42–46
    pre-stretched, 8–9
    recoil effects, 14, 45, 63, 71–72, 99–100
    reusability, 50
    selection of, 40–41
    terminology overview, 62–63
Kinesiology Taping applications
    contraindications, 30–33
    duration of application, 4, 53–54
    effects of, 13
    indications for, 26–29
    limits of, 13
    protection of, 33, 134
    removal of, 50–51, *50*
Knee joint
    case studies, 120–21, 126–28
    stabilization of, 103–4, *104–5*
Knee-Sling Taping, *4*, *21*

Lameness. *See* Gait abnormalities
Laser therapy, 54, 114, 133
Lateral, defined, *61*
Lifting effect
    benefits, 16, 28
    described, 14–15, *14*
    hair length and, *32*, 33
    signs of, 70
Ligament injuries, 3, 39, 126–27, 136–37
Long back muscle. *See M. Longissimus*
Lymphatic fluid/system, 16, 54, 74–75, *74*
Lymphatic Tapings
    overview, 80
    anchors for, 79–80, *80*
    application of, 75–77, *76–77*
    benefits, 31
    examples of, *23*

Fan-Tape cut for, 44

*M. latissimus dorsi*, 119–120
*M. Longissimus*
    about, 10, 67, *68*
    taping techniques for, 67–72, *69–70*, *72*
Magnetic blankets
    in case histories, 119, 120, 123, 131, 132, 137
    in conjunction with taping, 54
Malignancies, 31
Manual therapy
    in case studies, 118, 120, 123, 125
    in conjunction with taping, 54, 68
Massage
    in case studies, 118–126, 128–130, 132–34, 136–37
    in conjunction with taping, 13, 54, 68
    effects on fascia, 87–88
    for lymphatic drainage, 75
Mechanical receptor cells, 18
Medial, defined, *61*
Mobility, of joints, 15–16. *See also* Movement
Motion, study of, 6
Movement
    compensation for, 11
    of injured areas, 3
    range of motion, 16–17, 81
    taping effects, 39
Muscle belly, 66
Muscle memory, 3
Muscle Tapings
    application of, 45, 68–70
    for back, 67–73
    benefits, 27
    case studies, 119–122, 125–131, 134–37
    color effects in, 23
    requirements for, 66–67
    unilateral vs. bilateral, 73, *73*
Muscles
    activation/relaxation of, 13, 17, 26, 71–72, *72*
    atrophy of, 125–26
    injuries to, 3, 81
    pre-stretching of, 68
    problems in, 26
    support of, 17
    tension in, 15, 20, 23, 28

terminology for, 61–62
types of, 66–68
Myogelosis, 28, 62

Nerve cells, 87

Olympic Games, 2008, 5
Origin site, of muscles, 61, 66

Pain
  case studies, 129
  focal points of, 114
  taping for reduction of, 15–16, 29
Pain Cross. See Decompression Star Tapings
Paper backing, 46–47, 47
Patellar luxation, 127–28
Pelvis. See Hips
Physio tape, 7
Pink, color effects, 22
Positional terms, 60–61, 60–61
Precuts, 40
Pregnancy, as taping contraindication, 31
Preparation, 36
Pressure, reduction of, 15
Proprioception
  fascia role in, 17–18, 87, 110
  taping for improvement of, 17–18, 18, 26
Proprioception Tapings
  overview, 113
  application of, 52, 54, 110–13, 110, 112–13
  case studies, 18, 18, 119–120, 122–23, 136–37
  indications for, 110
Proximal, defined, 61
Purple, color effects, 22
Push-back. See Backup technique

Range of motion, 16–17, 81
Receptor cells, 8
Recoil effects
  overview, 14, 14, 63
  direction of, 71–72, 72
  in Stabilization Taping, 99–100
  tape application considerations, 45
Red, color effects, 20, 21
Relaxation, of muscles, 17, 26, 71–72, 72

Removal, of tapings, 50–51, 50
Reusability, 50
Row application, of Lymphatic Tapings, 78–79, 78

Sacrum/sacroiliac joint, 102, 102, 123–24
Scar Tapings
  overview, 86
  application of, 82–86, 83–86
  case studies, 124
  indications/contraindications, 28, 30
Scar tissue, 28, 30, 81–82, 82
Scissors, 45–46
Seasonal considerations, 50
"second skin," kinesiology tape as, 10–11, 26, 28
Sensory cells, 87
Shaped cuts, 43–44, 43–44
Sizing, of tape strips, 41
Skeletal musculature, 66–67
Skin
  air circulation for, 30
  diseases in, 30
  irritation risk, 31–32, 37, 52
  lifting effect and, 14, 32
  scar tissue, 28, 30, 81–82, 82
  static charge of, 114–15
  tape similar to, 10–11, 26, 28
Sling Tapings, 103–5, 104–5, 120–21
Smooth musculature, 66
Soft-tissue lesions, 3
Space Tape. See Decompression Star Tapings
Spasms, 62
Spine. See Back/spine
Spondylosis, 132
Sprains, 28, 29
Spray adhesives, 38
Spring back. See Recoil effects
Stabilization, of weak body parts, 3, 16–17
Stabilization Tapings
  overview, 102, 105
  benefits, 28
  case studies, 126–28, 132, 136–37
  examples of, 16
  for extremities, 103–5

indications for, 99
  for spine, 99–102
Star Tape. See Decompression Star Tapings
Static charge, of Cross Tapes, 114–15
Stress points, 114
Stretch, in tape applications, 49, 49, 51–52, 53, 93–94
Stretching exercises, 54, 121, 129
Support, taping for. See Stabilization Tapings
Supportive treatments, 13, 54–55, 59
Swelling, 15, 16, 27

Talcum powder, 38, 120
Tape, types of, 7. See also Kinesiology Tape
Tendon Tapings
  application of, 106–9, 106–9
  case studies, 121–22, 134–35
  color effects in, 23
  examples of, 29
Tendons
  function of, 66
  injuries to, 3, 28–29, 121–22
Term definitions, anatomical, 59–62
Tolerance, of animal for taping, 32–33, 52
Treatment modalities, combining taping with, 54–55
Trigger points, 28, 62, 92, 114
Tumors, 31, 124
Turquoise, color effects, 22

Ultrasound, 55
Unilateral tapings, 73

Ventral, defined, 60
Violet, color effects, 22
V-Tape cut. See Y-Tape cuts

Warming effects, 20, 23. See also Frictional heat, in activation of adhesive
Water, exposure of tape to, 54–55, 54
Wounds, 30, 31, 81

Yellow, color effects, 21
Y-Tape cuts, 43, 43, 89, 91